practice day in and day out. This book
many of my patients. . . . Many thanks f
nutritional aspects of people's health so
—Dr. Rae Lynn W

"I am thrilled that at last there is someone who is truly in tune with how we are feeling and that she doesn't want to prescribe some MEDICATION and say you will feel better soon. Hope at last. Thank you, thank you!!"

"I am SO excited to find this information!! For years I have racked my brain trying to figure out what made my son tick! . . . Also, my daughter has these INTENSE sugar cravings, particularly around her period. I have sent all your material to them. I KNOW this is the solution to both their problems. I certainly am going to apply some of it to myself. The three of us seem to have the same metabolism. Thank you so much!!!!!"
—T.W.

"FAB-ulous! . . . I've spent the last ten years experimenting with various foods trying to avoid "fuzz in the brain" along with emotional ups and downs. Your book finally explains it all."
—S.G.

"I loved the book. I couldn't put it down. . . . I feel like I've found what I have been searching for even though I didn't know what that was."
—N.B.

"Kathleen, you have my gratitude, respect and admiration! During the first four years of my sobriety from drugs and alcohol I gained over sixty pounds, telling myself that "at least it wasn't vodka" when I would microwave a nightly pint of Häagen-Dazs, or have a huge bowl of pasta for breakfast on weekends—now, six years and one child later, I have a commitment to both physical and emotional health and vigor—and the strong desire to see Nicholas reach his own adulthood without his mother constantly weeping, being couch-bound, or dead."
—T.

"Thank you, Kathleen DesMaisons!! Your book has been a godsend! . . . Through the entire book I was nodding my head, with tears streaming down my face, saying this is me, this is me." —D.K.

"Kathleen, thank you for writing your wonderful book. I am fifty-two and have had a "food" problem all my life. I have been on as many diets as there are in the world. I have always lost weight and always gained back more than I lost. I have suffered from the agony of knowing that I had no willpower, the agony of depression and the agony of worthlessness all my life. AND NEVER UNDERSTOOD WHY . . . I regard myself as a recovering alcoholic even though I took my sugar in a different form and thank God every day for this recovery. No more cravings. No more urges to eat the refrigerator. It's just a secondary thing, not a goal, but I have gone down three dress sizes since March 15 (my "D-day"). But that's not the important thing. Feeling like this for the rest of my life is the goal. Thank you, it's totally inadequate to say to you, because you gave me back my life, but it comes from the heart." —C.J.

Potatoes
Not Prozac

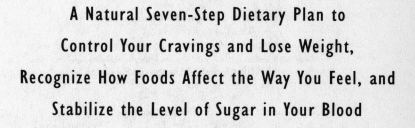

A Natural Seven-Step Dietary Plan to
Control Your Cravings and Lose Weight,
Recognize How Foods Affect the Way You Feel, and
Stabilize the Level of Sugar in Your Blood

Kathleen DesMaisons, Ph.D.

A Fireside Book
Published by Simon & Schuster

FIRESIDE
Rockefeller Center
1230 Avenue of the Americas
New York, NY 10020

First Fireside Edition 1999

FIRESIDE and colophon are registered trademarks
of Simon & Schuster Inc.

Designed by Chris Welch

Manufactured in the United States of America

1   3   5   7   9   10   8   6   4   2

Library of Congress Cataloging-in-Publication Data
DesMaisons, Kathleen.
Potatoes not prozac : a natural seven-step dietary plan to control your cravings and
lose weight, recognize how foods affect the way you feel, and stabilize the level of
sugar in your blood/Kathleen DesMaisons—1st Fireside ed.
p.   cm.
"A Fireside book."
Includes bibliographical references and index.
1. Sugar-free diet   2. Compulsive eating—Diet therapy.   3. Compulsive eating
—Psychosomatic aspects.   4. Depression, Mental—Diet therapy.   5. Depression,
Mental—Psychosomatic aspects.   6. Reducing diets   I. Title.
RM237.85.D47   1999
613.2'5—dc21   98-48491
                                                                          CIP

ISBN 0-684-84953-4
0-684-85014-1 (Pbk)

The recommendations in this book are not intended to replace or conflict with advice given
to you by your physician or other health care professional. If you have any preexisting medical
or psychological conditions, or if you are currently taking medication, you should consult with
your physician before adopting the suggestions and procedures in this book. Following these
dietary suggestions may impact the effect of certain types of medication. Any changes in your
dosage should be made only in cooperation with your prescribing physician.

Prozac is a trademark of Eli Lilly and Company. This book is not affiliated with or authorized
by Eli Lilly and Company.

To Mother, who demanded that this story be told and who guided every step of the way. Let me always remember that this is really your work.

Acknowledgments

Moving from the dream of a book to the finished product is a big process. Many people have helped to make this vision real. It started in the rooms of courageous men and women who had tried everything and still felt terrible. Their quest for recovery moved me to my own. The shared journey led to the reality of the story now being told in this way.

Thank you to the Union Institute who gave me the freedom to create a doctoral program which could go as deep and as rigorously as I hoped. Thanks to Ira Fritz, my advisor there, who believed in me from the beginning. Christina Gianoulakis and Elliott Blass, mouse doctors par excellence, trusted and cheered me to rigorous and imaginative thought. Tammy Ramirez convinced me that statistics could be fun and helped me to loosen up and have fun with my numbers.

Deberah Bringelson convinced the Peninsula Foundation that food for drunk drivers was not just some woo-woo California idea. Judge Craig Parsons, Janice McLaren and Pat Pritchard made it happen. Peggy Thompson put all the systems in place and has steadfastly oiled the gears so there has never been even a squeak. Michael Nevins, John Maltbie, Margaret Taylor and Don Horsley believed enough to make the program a part of the County system. My dedicated staff, George Forrester, Rita Tovar and Katherine Alden, have kept the fires burning through all those days and nights that I sat at the computer writing.

Christiane Northrop's unabashed enthusiasm started the publishing miracle you now hold. I thank her for recognizing the power of the story and standing with me in finding a home for the book. Special thanks to a visionary and gifted agent, Ned Leavitt, who ran with the manuscript so well I had to run to keep up. I am honored to be represented by a man of such skill and integrity.

The Simon & Schuster family is a home which fits perfectly all I hoped for in a publisher. Carolyn Reidy's leadership sets a remarkable tone for balancing risk-taking with careful hard work. My editor, Mary Ann Naples, understood the heart of this story and knew immediately what it could mean for so many people. Her humor, grace and skill represent the best of professionalism. Every staff member I have worked with reflects pride and commitment.

Special thanks to my three children and their father who cheered me on and held steadfast in trusting that I could really write a book. Their support and encouragement nurtured me through the hard times. Their belief was mirrored by dear friends who supported me all the way. I am grateful for Debbra Colman's encouragement and prayers, which have always been steady as a rock, Chris Ortega's listening at every step along the way, Joel Wheeler's affirmation of a horrible first draft which made it possible to write another, and Margo Silk-Forrest's teaching the craft of writing which could speak my knowing.

And last but not least, thanks to Vancouver D. Dawg, the guide-dog-in-training who got up with me every morning before dawn to lie at my feet while I tapped into the computer. Vancouver has taught me that love and service can go hand in hand to make wonderful things happen.

Contents

Foreword

While we think of sugar as a food, it is actually a drug—an external substance acting throughout the brain and body on cellular receptors designed for an internal chemical called glucose. Since glucose is usually the only fuel the brain can ever use, and is critical to mental clarity, mood states and the controlled release of energy in the body, it is astounding how cavalierly we sprinkle sugar, its inferior substitute, into everything from children's breakfast food to ketchup. If sugar were to be put on the market for the first time today, it would probably be difficult to get it past the FDA.

Like many drugs that work through receptors, sugar has a paradoxical effect characterized by two phenomena: First, the more of the drug you take, the less of the drug's internal analog is produced in your brain and body. Second, the receptors for sugar or any other drug become less sensitive—sometimes actually decreasing in number—as protection against the drug bombarding them. We can easily become physically dependent on exogenous sugar for mood boosts—but our habit now results in depression instead of well-being, exhaustion and anxiety instead of a burst of energy. I have long suspected that the increase of clinical depression in our society is linked to the increased consumption of sugar.

How exciting it was for me, then, to hear about Kathleen Des-Maisons's efforts in developing a working hypothesis about sugar sensitivity and its role in addictive behavior. I have been aware of her work for many years. Her vision, personal warmth and passionate commitment to finding answers have always touched me. *Potatoes Not Prozac* now moves her vision into concrete, specific guidance that brings her clinical skills to a wider audience.

Dr. DesMaisons has a unique gift for taking very complex ideas and making them accessible for regular folks who are trying to feel better. Her thesis is persuasive. Her combination of clinical experience, personal honesty and scientific curiosity have led to real benefits for her clients. While the stories remain anecdotal from a scientific perspective, they are powerful to hear. As Dr. DesMaisons suggests, something is going on in the relationship between diet and behavior —something beyond what scientific research has already shown about biochemistry and mood.

As a scientist I could never entertain that the size of my childhood trick-or-treat bag at Halloween could have any meaning. But as a woman who has struggled with some of the problems Dr. DesMaisons talks about, I would not be so quick to dismiss her ideas. Sometimes science is nudged by pioneers from the field who put studies together in new ways and ask questions from an unexpected perspective. The scientific story will be tested in the laboratory. But the day-to-day impact of *Potatoes Not Prozac* will be tested in the hearts and bodies of the people who identify with the profile Dr. DesMaisons has so powerfully outlined.

Foods can act as drugs, and we must be aware of how our moods and physiology—mental and physical—are so inextricably intertwined that what and how we eat can have an enormous impact on our lives. I highly recommend *Potatoes Not Prozac*, which I believe contains novel and important information for everyone from the most sophisticated nutritionist to the individual who is just beginning to realize that what and how we eat helps to explain why we feel the way we feel.

Candace B. Pert, Ph.D.
Author of *Molecules of Emotion: Why We Feel the Way We Feel*
Research Professor
Department of Physiology and Biophysics
Georgetown University Medical Center

Chapter 1

✦

Dr. Jekyll and Mr. Hyde

Are you aware of yourself, smart and sensitive to others' feelings? Are you committed to your own personal growth? Do you care about things deeply? Do your friends value you and respect your opinion? Are you successful in your work? Are you usually confident and hopeful about your future?

But do you sometimes feel your confidence slip away, leaving you in self-doubt and despair? Does it seem "crazy" that you can be so clear one day and so desperate the next? Worse, you may drop from the heights to the depths in the same day. It's almost as if another person were inside you.

You hate to admit it, but you can be moody and impulsive. You want to get things done, but your attention drifts. You lose energy and get tired. You crave sugar and turn to sweets and snack foods to get yourself going again. Sometimes you eat compulsively. You put on weight. You seem to have no self-discipline. You often feel depressed and overwhelmed.

You may have consulted your doctor. You may have gotten counseling from your pastor or a psychotherapist. You may have been put on Prozac or one of the other antidepressants. But something is still wrong. Your life is still not the way you want it to be and you can't seem to find an answer that works.

If this description fits you, you may be sugar sensitive. Your body chemistry may respond to sugars and certain carbohydrates (such as bread, crackers, cereal and pasta) differently than other people's. This biochemical difference can have a huge effect on your moods and your behavior. How you feel is linked to what you eat—and when you eat it.

Listen to Emily's story:

I was overweight, depressed and exhausted all the time. I had a lot to be grateful for in my life, but something was wrong. Why didn't I feel better about myself? Why was my battle with those extra twenty pounds so hopeless? Why didn't I have the energy to do more in life? I was so discouraged.

I drank several cups of coffee a day, snacked on gummy bears, and ate healthy foods like pasta, vegetables and fruits. I avoided fats and high-calorie desserts. Sometimes I grazed throughout the day, sometimes I'd skip meals and eat only once a day. Although I had tried lots of diets, I always regained the weight I lost. I would start an exercise program, stick to it for a few weeks, then go off my diet and stop exercising. I still was overweight and hating it. I felt like a failure in this part of my life and I was ashamed of it.

Often I couldn't sleep and I was plagued by anxious feelings. Sometimes my heart would start racing for no reason. I had sudden outbursts of crying or anger. I tried therapy, figuring I was just "not right." But it wasn't enough.

So I went to my doctor and told her my long list of problems. She looked concerned and ordered a series of exams. I too was concerned. Maybe I was starting menopause early. I even worried I might have a brain tumor. A week later my doctor called. "I have good news and bad news," she told me. "The good news is that you are not in menopause and you don't have a brain tumor. The bad news is that I don't know what is happening. Your lab tests and your physical exam results are all normal."

Frustrated and depressed, Emily came into my private practice in Addictive Nutrition. She told me she was a recovering alcoholic with nine years of successful sobriety and had heard that I was using nutrition to help people with her symptoms. After listening to her story and asking her some questions about her background and her eating habits, I recognized what was wrong. I had seen it time and again in women and men seeking help for compulsive eating, alcoholism, drug addiction or this strange collection of symptoms that had not responded to other treatments.

Emily was neither clinically depressed nor suffering from the effects of a bad childhood. She was not weak-willed or lazy. She was sugar sensitive. Emily had a special kind of body chemistry that made her more vulnerable to the mood-altering effects of sweet foods and refined-flour products than her friends were. She was caught in a vicious cycle of highs and lows controlled by her blood sugar levels and her brain chemicals. Emily responded to sugar as if it were a drug.

Sugar Sensitivity

Sugar sensitivity turns a person into Dr. Jekyll and Mr. Hyde. It's like having two different people live in your body. From one moment to the next your fine sensitivity and openness turn into moodiness and irritability. Your confidence and creativity dry up, only to be replaced by low self-esteem and hopelessness. Your visions for the future dissipate into the frustration born of not following through.

This emotional Ping-Pong remains inexplicable without an understanding of sugar sensitivity. Like Emily, millions of people who have sugar-sensitive bodies are caught in the pain of not understanding a problem that controls their lives. Sugar-sensitive people seem to know instinctively that something is wrong but cannot make sense of what it is.

Do you feel this way? If so, your intuition may be right on target. If you are sugar sensitive you are not inherently weak-willed or without self-discipline. Your behavior reflects a skewed body chemistry which you have tried to correct unconsciously by self-medicating with sugars and carbohydrates.

Your sugar sensitivity is a problem that you inherited. You did not create this dilemma. It is not your fault. What's more, it is a problem that can be solved. I have an answer that you have been seeking for a long time. Clear and simple, the solution to sugar sensitivity makes perfect sense. As you begin to understand how your blood sugar levels and brain chemicals work and interact, you will start to appreciate the power of your own body. Instead of being driven by your body chemistry, you will begin to chart your own life. You will find a straightforward explanation for the behavior you have struggled with for so long—and a straightforward solution based on giving your body the kinds of foods it needs to keep your emotions in balance and your life in forward gear.

This book tells the story of sugar sensitivity.

Naming the Problem

The story of sugar sensitivity comes out of my own personal history and my work with thousands of clients in addiction treatment. After a long career in public health I started an addiction treatment center in 1988 because I wanted to make a difference in people's lives. The typical recovery rate for alcoholism is dismally low. People relapse. People relapse again—and again and again. Although addiction experts have tried many alternatives, the picture remains pretty grim. A 25 percent success rate is considered good. But accepting not being able to help three out of every four people who came into my clinic was out of the question for me. I knew there had to be a better way —and I set out to find it.

My determination to beat the odds comes out of my personal history. When I was sixteen my father died of alcoholism at the age of fifty-one. He was a brilliant, sensitive man who couldn't find his way out of the bottle. They say he loved to party as a young man; by the time he reached middle age he was drinking a fifth of vodka every day.

My father stayed sober for one year, the year I turned eleven. He was a career officer in the Air Force and his superiors had threatened to discharge him from the service if he didn't stop drinking. So he went into detox and rehabilitation for the first—and only—time. I remember that year well. With my father sober, life was so much better for all of us. Everything I had secretly dreamed of was happening and we finally lived like a normal family.

One year later, despite being sober, my father was discharged from the Air Force for alcoholism. Past job evaluations had followed him and the Air Force did not recognize—or perhaps did not believe—his commitment to sobriety. In losing his job, my father was cut from his lifeline. His sobriety and our family's newfound stability careened rapidly downhill. Five years later he was dead.

It took me twenty-five years to grieve the loss of my father. At the time I felt only relief—relief that I no longer had to be ashamed of his drinking. All I wanted then was a normal teenage life. After Dad's death, we all colluded in creating a family myth that he had died suddenly of pancreatitis. In reality, he had been dying of alcoholism for five years, but not one of us ever talked about it. We just carried on, folding our wounds into the tapestry of our lives, each trying to make sense of the tragedy alone.

"Don't Tell. Don't Feel. Don't Share."

My history has shaped me deeply. Because of my father's alcoholic behavior I learned to pay close attention to the interpersonal dynamics around me. I learned to immediately "read" the emotional temperature of almost any situation. I learned to grow up early, become a high achiever, be the hero in my family. Most of all, I learned the inviolable rules of an alcoholic family:

"Don't tell. Don't feel. Don't share."

"What you see isn't really happening."

"Everything is fine, even though you feel something else."

I learned to live in dissonance. I kept confronting the discrepancy between what the folks around me said was true and what I experienced in my body and in my heart. I challenged my mother about the lies of our family life. I challenged my religion teachers about the difference between what the church said and how people acted. I constantly asked questions about the gap between the ideal and the real. I studied everything I could to try to find a solution for the dilemma of this discrepancy. I wanted to live what I believed and I wanted the world to do the same.

At nineteen, still dreaming of the perfect family, I married and had three babies in rapid succession. But the gap between my ideal life and my real life still loomed large. Although smart and successful both in school and as a new parent, I was overweight and subject to extreme mood swings and sudden drops in energy. Sometimes I was filled with self-confidence and felt clear and focused. At other times I would drift into a sort of "la-la land" and forget to buy milk for the children. My husband thought he'd married Dr. Jekyll and ended up getting Ms. Hyde, too. He wondered how my behavior could change so quickly. As for me, I didn't really notice my own behavior. I was well trained to overlook dysfunction, including my own.

My marriage stopped working when my youngest child was six months old. Neither my young husband nor I knew how to make a relationship work or how to ask for help. Single again, I returned to college, worked full-time and threw myself into the task of raising my children. In the evening, after I had put everyone to bed, I sat on the couch with Coke and popcorn, reading philosophy and folding laundry.

When I was twenty-six I came down with mononucleosis, which damaged my liver. Because my liver was impaired, alcohol made me sick, so I stopped drinking. It was a straightforward decision, but it probably saved my life. As with most children of alcoholics, I was a sitting duck for alcoholism. My body chemistry was primed to need alcohol, and had I kept drinking I would have gone from enjoyment to dependence to abuse.

Turning to Sugar for Solace

But abstinence from alcohol nudged me onto a different path of addiction. Alcohol hadn't hooked me, but sugar, ice cream, pasta, bread and soda did. These seemingly harmless foods wrapped me in a cocoon so thick and numbing that I never missed the alcohol.

When I finished college I went on to complete a master's degree in management and counseling. The high-achieving child of an alcoholic that I was, I was hired as the director of a nonprofit program before I even finished my degree. Eighteen months later I was promoted to supervise a hundred staff members. On the outside I appeared successful, competent and skilled. On the inside I was running from my own feelings. I sensed a huge pool of pain swirling below the bravado. I wasn't aware of the impact of my father's alcoholism on me and I hadn't a clue about what was driving my life.

Finally, at the age of thirty, I could no longer ignore my pain. I realized I needed help and I went into therapy. Because I was the head of a community mental-health center, I thought I should maintain the appearance of being emotionally "together." So I traveled two hours and a hundred miles each way every week to see my therapist. She encouraged me to express my anger. "I won't," I would say. "Anger kills. It isn't safe." For a whole year we argued. Finally I let myself go and got angry. But my anger was directed not at my father or my family—it was directed at my therapist. I was angry about the direction of my therapy and the dissonance I felt between what she was saying and what she was doing. Two days later she committed suicide. It was hard for me to understand that her death was not my fault. I was just thirty and no one even knew I had been in therapy. "Don't tell," "don't feel" and "don't share" still drove my response to pain.

I didn't have the skills to make sense of the pain so I turned to doughnuts, a new town and a new job. Perhaps a new life would make things better. I moved to a place near the ocean. I was comforted by the sea. I lived next door to an ice cream parlor. I was comforted by the ice cream. I gained more weight. The early pattern my ex-husband had identified continued. I was still Dr. Jekyll and Ms. Hyde. When I was good I was very, very good, and when I wasn't, I fell apart. I tried hard to hold it all together, but when I hit forty I realized that my life would unravel if I didn't try again to face my pain. The old gap between my inner feelings and my external life had stretched to the limit.

My solution then was to move to California, where the softness of the hills, the sound of the sea and the openness of the people all soothed me. I reconnected to the child within me who loved to swim and dance and laugh. I started feeling good about myself, but my weight and my mood swings continued to plague me. After every diet I gained back the weight I'd lost. Because I thought my problem with food had its roots in emotional wounding, I worked on my inner development for years. I read hundreds of books, attended dozens of groups and seminars, and filled countless journals with poetry.

No matter how much inner work I did, though, I seemed to be fighting a losing battle. The needle on my bathroom scale was now nearing 240, but I thought the problem was just a matter of willpower. When I developed enough discipline, everything would be fine. As time went on and things didn't change, I lived with deeper and deeper feelings of inadequacy.

Lessons from the "Drunks"

In spite of—or perhaps because of—an inner sense of hopelessness, I continued to be committed to helping others heal. I was asked by the county I worked in to start a treatment center for alcoholics and drug addicts. To me, the idea of doing this work felt like "coming home" and I leapt at the chance. Once the clinic got going I found myself frequently abandoning my desk to work directly with our clients. The alcoholics who came into our clinic mirrored both my father's story and my own. They were trying to keep their lives from crumbling beneath them.

Although I had spent twenty years working in public health, I only really began to get it about alcoholism and drug addiction when I heard these people's halting voices and listened to their painful stories. What I learned was that what we were doing—counseling, support groups and pleas for abstinence—didn't work particularly well. Even "good" treatment done by sensitive, caring and trained professionals didn't help much. Our clients kept relapsing despite their best intentions to "work the program." Our recovery rate was no better than the national average. I needed to find out why.

The more I listened to the "drunks," the more I was struck by some missing link between what I heard them say and what I felt. I knew in my heart that their addiction to alcohol was not about a lack of willpower. I knew drinking wasn't just an easy way out to escape unpleasant feelings. Something else was going on. I was convinced that if I discovered this missing link our treatment program for alcoholism might succeed.

At the same time there was a troubling discrepancy between my work at the clinic and my own life. Although I hadn't used alcohol in eighteen years, I had never been in any kind of recovery program. I didn't see my compulsive use of food, particularly sugars and carbohydrates, as an addiction. I just thought I was fat and that this was a function of my early childhood issues. A thousand failed diets had convinced me that I was a slug who couldn't get it right. Since I was successful on the outside, I hid my feelings of despair and put in even longer hours.

Yet as I worked with alcoholics and drug addicts, I started being drawn subtly into recovery. At moments, I wished I were an alcoholic myself so I could put words to my own suffering. I didn't have a name for my story then, but I began to see that I was going to have to live out the ideas I was teaching. I didn't want to just teach recovery, I wanted to have it.

This meant I had to confront my past. So I started learning what it meant to be the child of an alcoholic, what it meant to be codependent, and how playing the role of the hero—taking responsibility for others' needs instead of my own—had shaped my professional development. My ending up in charge of an alcoholism treatment center, surrounded by a "bunch of drunks," was no accident. By the grace of something much bigger than myself, I stayed with the process —working on myself while I worked with the men and women at my clinic.

Discovering Food as Pharmacy

My recovery focused on using the Twelve Steps which originated in Alcoholics Anonymous and started with the idea of surrender to a "higher power." The idea of surrendering to a higher power didn't work for me. But surrendering to something "deeper" did. So I handed my life over to the something deeper and asked for help. One day, by chance, a friend told me that she had been following a food plan that had really worked for her. She was eating protein and vegetables. I tried it and started losing weight, which surprised and pleased me. But even more astounding was what happened to my moods and behavior. I didn't crave sweet things. I didn't dream about bread and pasta. My emotional ups and downs evened out. I wasn't confused or foggy at certain times in the day. I was able to think clearly. I got things done. I set goals and moved toward them without a constant struggle to stay focused.

Although I had done a lot of work on my inner self, I knew the changes I was experiencing were not psychological. They were *physiological*. I hadn't suddenly gotten my act together. Something had happened in my brain and in my body, and it felt like the missing link I'd been searching for. I had changed my food—mostly by cutting down on sugars and starches—and subsequently experienced a huge change in my physical and emotional well-being. I began to wonder whether, being the child of an alcoholic, I had inherited an alcoholic's body chemistry. Perhaps alcoholics and compulsive eaters like me are hypersensitive to sugar. Perhaps my body physiologically craved sugar the same way my father's body had physiologically craved alcohol. If so, I thought, wouldn't this hold true for my clients as well?

So I went to my clients. Asking these men and women what kinds of foods they ate revealed data that was no surprise to me. My clients' eating habits closely resembled my own previous eating patterns. No wonder I felt such an affiliation with these "drunks"! Almost none of them ate breakfast, few ate regular meals, most ate a very high percentage of white bread, pasta and cereal, and all ate a great many sweets. Whenever I talked to clients who were unable to stay sober, I found they were eating primarily sweet things and refined-flour products.

Almost immediately I added nutritional awareness as one of my clinic's steps to recovery. I put together a food plan for sugar-sensitive people, a plan based on protein, complex carbohydrates (like whole wheat, potatoes and brown rice), fruit and vegetables. The food plan was simple, easy and affordable. The plan I developed filled in the gaps I had experienced in my friend's program when I had used it myself. I intuitively knew that eating only protein and vegetables wasn't the best alternative—our bodies need more carbohydrates on an ongoing basis than her plan provided. But if I kept the basic concept, added *complex* carbohydrates and continued to minimize the use of sugars, I was sure the revised food plan would work. I also added an educational component directed at the addictive personalities of my clients.

I told my clients that this food plan was not a diet but a way of eating for life. I explained to them my theory about sugar sensitivity and how it might be predisposing them to alcoholism. When I told them that eating sugar could sabotage their recovery from addiction by priming them to crave alcohol, they sat up and paid attention. Then they tried the food plan—and got remarkable results.

As my clients changed their diets, their lives began to improve in a number of ways. Compared to other clients we had seen at the clinic, their withdrawal symptoms passed more quickly and gave them less discomfort. Their mood swings mellowed. Their cravings diminished. Their energy increased. They were more enthusiastic and committed to their recovery than ever. People who had never been able to achieve sobriety began getting—and staying—sober.

After using the food plan with several hundred men and women, I found we were achieving unusual success with alcoholics and drug addicts. The track record told me it was time to establish a scientific basis for the changes I saw coming from my food plan. I decided to leave my job and sell my house to start working on my Ph.D.

Finding Out Why It Worked

My doctoral research took me into professional journals and academic textbooks on nutrition, endocrinology, psychopharmacology, psychiatry and addiction. I learned about the wide-ranging effects of blood sugar and the powerful emotional impact of certain brain chemicals, chemicals which can get pushed out of balance by an overuse of sugar.

One of these brain chemicals, serotonin, was becoming better known to the public, thanks to the advent of Prozac, the new antidepressant that boosts serotonin levels and brings feelings of optimism, creativity and peace of mind. To my astonishment, the other brain chemical I was learning about, beta-endorphin, was as critical to emotional well-being as serotonin but was not being discussed outside scientific circles. My reading showed me that beta-endorphin has a direct impact on a person's self-esteem, tolerance for pain (including emotional pain), sense of connectedness to others and ability to take personal responsibility for action. You'll learn all about this amazing brain chemical later in the book. For now, let's go back to my story.

As I worked on my doctorate I found that all of the biochemical facts I was learning fit with my clinical results to form an elegant and compelling story. My research confirmed my suspicions—and the name I had given to that story. Sugar sensitivity has a basis in rigorous science. I was amazed that no one was telling the public about it.

For my doctoral dissertation I conducted a study to measure the effect of my food plan on the toughest audience I could find—multiple-offender drunk drivers. These people—mostly middle-aged men —had not been able to stay sober despite huge court sanctions and intensive drunk-driving education and counseling. All of them had already gone through an entire forty-hour first offender program, had paid thousands of dollars in fines and fees, and had now lost their driver's licenses for eighteen months. I worked with a group of thirty of these "hopeless" alcoholics for four months and at the end of my outpatient treatment program, 92 percent of them had gotten sober and stayed sober. These clients weren't drinking and for the first time in their lives they were experiencing recovery. Eighteen months later I checked back with them and only a few were back to serious drinking. The rest maintained their sobriety or had significantly reduced the level of their drinking. These same results continue as the program has grown to serve close to two hundred people.

In addition, my success with sugar sensitivity went far beyond helping people to stop drinking. At the same time I was working with drunk drivers, my private practice was filled with women and men who were overweight or ate compulsively, adult children of alcoholics who felt tired, crazy and depressed, and former addicts and alcoholics who, though clean and sober, still didn't feel well.

I became known as "the lady of last resort." When people had tried everything and still felt rotten, they came to me. I explained to them how their blood sugar, serotonin and beta-endorphin worked and showed them how to use my food plan. When they tried it, these people experienced the same miraculous shift that my drunk drivers and I had experienced. Not surprisingly, word began to get out. More and more people from across the country called me for help. I promised I would write a book about sugar sensitivity and the crucial role of beta-endorphin.

Potatoes Not Prozac is that book. It offers you a simple program for counteracting the effects of sugar sensitivity and shows you how to make that miraculous shift happen in your own life. What's more, you will be able to do this without going on another deprivation diet. You will not have to throw away the foods you love. You will not have to make radical changes that drive you crazy.

The seven-step program you'll learn is a gentle, simple process that respects your style and your needs. You will be able to read your body and design a food plan that works for you. During this process I will help you understand the "why" of feelings you have never been able to resolve. You will come to understand what you have known intuitively but been unable to name. You will find an answer you have been looking for.

Potatoes Not Prozac is for every child of an alcoholic and every man and woman who is tired of looking good on the outside while feeling bad inside. It is for everyone stuck in addiction, depression, low self-esteem and compulsive behavior. This book is my story and it is your story. It is the story of all of us who have waited so long and tried so hard to get free of these "crazy" feelings and our Dr. Jekyll/ Mr. Hyde behaviors. One powerful answer is biochemical. One answer is sugar sensitivity.

Chapter 2

✦

Are You Sugar Sensitive?

By now you are probably wondering if you, too, are sugar sensitive. And if so, how sugar sensitive are you?

There are two ways to determine this, both of which I use with my clients. Some people prefer the informal approach, others like using the checklist and questionnaire included later in this chapter. Let's start with an informal way to diagnose sugar sensitivity. When a client comes to see me about compulsive eating, I start by asking a simple question.

> Imagine you come home and go into the kitchen. A plate of warm chocolate-chip cookies sits on the counter just out of the oven. Their smell hits you as you walk in. You do not feel hungry. No one else is around. What would you do?

Does this question make you smile? You may think the answer is obvious, but people who are not sugar sensitive respond by saying, "Why would I eat a cookie if I wasn't hungry?" Or they stop and think about whether they would eat the cookie. Or, with no emotional charge, they say, "Well, I might try one." People who are not sugar sensitive do not have a visceral response to the idea of smelling fresh chocolate-chip cookies.

People who *are* sugar sensitive laugh at the cookie question. Their bodies are already responding to the very idea of the cookies. They know they would inhale a cookie—probably more than one, at that!

They might eat the whole plateful, even if they were not hungry. For a sugar-sensitive person, hunger is not the driving motivation. What triggers their desire to eat is the smell of the cookies, the anticipation of how the cookies will feel in the mouth, and the warmth and sweetness of the chocolate. Even the feeling of having a cookie in hand will have a powerful association for them. Those cookies mean love, they mean comfort. The cookies are friends and lovers.

People who are not sugar sensitive think this response to the cookies is strange, perhaps even stupid: "What on earth are you talking about?" But people who are sugar sensitive always know exactly what the cookie question means.

I have asked this question of many, many groups. Every time I've received dramatically consistent responses. While one part of the group will be waiting for the punch line after I ask, "Would you eat a cookie?" all the sugar-sensitive people are laughing. Their bodies were already responding to the image of the plate full of warm cookies in the kitchen. Try this experiment with your friends and see what kind of response you get.

A second powerful diagnostic question that I use is this:

When you were little and had Rice Krispies for breakfast, did you eat the cereal or did you eat the cereal so you could get to the milk and sugar at the bottom of the bowl?

People who are not sugar sensitive think the milk and sugar at the bottom of the bowl are disgusting. People who *are* sugar sensitive smile. They remember that the real objective was to get to the dregs of milk and sugar. They got high by tilting the cereal bowl into their mouths and tasting the clump of sugar at the bottom.

Your answers to these two questions may simply reinforce what you already know. Some people—perhaps including you—are very attached to sweet things.

There are lots of other ways to get clues to your sugar sensitivity. You might think back to the size of the bag you carried at Halloween. Children who were not sugar sensitive carried those small orange plastic pumpkins. We carried pillowcases. Their candy lasted until Easter. Ours was gone in three days.

Diagnosing Sugar Sensitivity

If you are still asking, How can I know for sure if I am sugar sensitive? let's take a look at the core issues associated with sugar sensitivity. Check each of the statements that applies to you:

> ❑   I really like sweet foods.
>
> ❑   I eat a lot of sweets.
>
> ❑   I am very fond of bread, cereal, popcorn, or pasta.
>
> ❑   I now have or have had a problem with alcohol or drugs.
>
> ❑   One or both of my parents are/were alcoholic.
>
> ❑   One or both of my parents are/were especially fond of sugar.
>
> ❑   I am overweight and don't seem to be able to easily lose the extra pounds.
>
> ❑   I continue to be depressed no matter what I do.
>
> ❑   I often find myself overreacting to stress.
>
> ❑   I have a history of anger that sometimes surprises even me.

How many boxes did you check? If you checked three or more, you are reading the right book. If you checked all ten, you are in good company. Each of these statements relates to an aspect of sugar sensitivity. Let's go through them one at a time so you can see what your answers may have to tell you.

I really like sweet foods.

Answering yes to this question alone indicates sugar sensitivity. If you *really* like sweet foods, you may have an intense physiological response to them. Sugar-sensitive people actually respond to tasting and eating sugar in a way that is more pronounced than other people's. A "normal" person will enjoy sweets, but can eat half a cookie and leave the rest for tomorrow. A "normal" person doesn't sit through dinner thinking about dessert. A "normal" person does not feel more confident and powerful after eating sweet things.

I eat a lot of sweets.

Sugar-sensitive people are likely to eat a lot of sweets. Even though you feel you shouldn't, you may eat candy, cookies or ice cream. Dessert may be the most important part of your meal. You may not eat sweet things during the day and then binge at night.

Or you may really love sweet things but choose not to eat them. Lindsay, a tall, slender client of mine, was sugar sensitive. Because she was concerned about calories and fats in her diet, she had stopped eating hot fudge sundaes, candy bars and the other sweets she usually craved. But even though she had eliminated obvious sugars from her diet, sweet things continued to find their way into her mouth. She ate power bars for breakfast. She stopped drinking Coke and switched to fruit juice. She also discovered she loved carrot juice. She would have a glass of wine with dinner as a treat to make up for how much she missed her high-calorie splurges.

But all of these foods contain high amounts of sugar. Lindsay's biochemistry was craving sugars and drove her to find them even without her knowing what she was doing. Her power bars and many of the other "healthy" low-fat foods she ate were very high in what their labels called carbohydrates. Sugars come in many forms. People who are sugar sensitive find them. Go to page 120 for a fuller discussion of sugars.

I am very fond of bread, cereal, popcorn or pasta.

Your body may respond to foods made with white flour as if they were sugars. You may find you feel good soon after eating them but then feel terrible later on. You may love bread. Cereal may be a staple for you. In the evening, you might settle on the couch with a huge bowl of popcorn.

Rank yourself on a scale of 1 to 10 on your attachment to any of these foods. You may be surprised to find that even though you don't eat "sugar," you have a very powerful emotional attachment to bread, cereal, popcorn or pasta. You would kill for French bread. You know where all the homemade pasta is sold. Don't get nervous. It's okay to feel this way. Your attachment to these foods tells us only how powerful your sugar-sensitive biochemistry is.

I now have or have had a problem with alcohol or drugs.

If you have used alcohol or drugs in an addictive way at some time in your life, it's very likely that you have a body chemistry that responds more intensely to alcohol or drugs than other people's. Your attachment to sugars sets you up biochemically for the addictive use of alcohol and even certain drugs.

Even if you are recovering from alcohol or drug addiction, sugar sensitivity can affect how you feel. This accounts for much of the syndrome called the dry drunk. Hair-trigger reactions and impulsive behavior can be caused by what you eat and when you eat it. Many of the unexplained physical and emotional symptoms that people take for granted in addiction recovery, such as irritability, cravings, mood swings and sleep disturbances, actually result from having a sugar-sensitive body. In addition, feelings of low self-esteem may continue long after they seem rationally warranted. For example, Christine, who got sober five years ago, expected to feel a whole lot happier and healthier than she does. She has a fabulous job, which she loves, has been promoted three times in two years and makes $20,000 more a year, but still worries that she will be a bag lady in her old age. The problem is that Christine stopped drinking but didn't change her diet to compensate for her sugar-sensitive body. What and when you eat can make you feel terrible or wonderful.

One or both of my parents are/were alcoholic.

If your parents drank to excess or drank in an alcoholic fashion, you may have inherited a specific type of brain-chemical response to alcohol that makes you feel tearful, depressed and emotionally overwhelmed—or angry and belligerent—when you are under the influence. You can inherit other aspects of sugar sensitivity as well. Your parents may have been sugar sensitive long before they started to drink. Seventy-eight percent of the drunk drivers in the program I ran reported that their fathers were alcoholics and their mothers loved sweets. This combination of an alcoholic father and a sugar-sensitive mother, or vice versa, maximizes the chance that you were born with a sugar-sensitive body.

One or both of my parents are/were especially fond of sugar.

People who are sugar sensitive often grow up in houses where sweets abound. I remember our family ritual of going to the local Dairy Queen on summer evenings. Ice cream not only created a pleasant memory, it carried a whole emotional charge as well. To this day, the memory of the sweet, cold, creamy soft treat evokes a powerful and pleasant response in my body.

As with the question about chocolate-chip cookies, non-sugar-sensitive people do not respond in this way. They may report a childhood memory of going to Dairy Queen, but it's a memory with a different emotional content. Their bodies do not remember the feeling of the ice cream in their mouths with the same intensity. Ask a non-sugar-sensitive person what he or she remembers about food from childhood. Then ask a sugar-sensitive person. I guarantee there will be a big difference in their responses.

I am overweight and don't seem to be able to easily lose the extra pounds.

Sugar-sensitive people often crave carbohydrates. This isn't an emotional craving but a physiological one caused by the way their body chemistry overreacts to eating sweets and carbohydrates. They find dieting difficult and often unproductive in the long term. Restricting calories does not result in weight loss as it should. People who are sugar sensitive can eat as few as 800 calories a day, and if those calories are from carbohydrates they will still gain weight. They may have tried a high-protein diet, like that recommended in Barry Sears's *Mastering the Zone*, and initially had success. But over time it is likely that they started feeling restless and uneasy. Then they slipped and ate carbohydrates, could not get back on the diet and experienced a disastrous rebound effect. You know the "yo-yo syndrome" well: lose ten pounds, regain fifteen; lose fifteen, regain twenty.

I continue to be depressed no matter what I do.

Sugar-sensitive people may have a hard time getting mobilized. You may feel frequently sad or apathetic. You may be depressed and crawl through the day with very little energy. For women, the depression may get worse just before menstruation. Often, sugar-sensitive people are miserable in the winter because the decrease in daylight affects their already impaired brain chemicals. You may self-medicate your depression by eating sweet foods since sweets are one of the few things that make you feel better. You may be taking an antidepressant like Prozac but still have symptoms of depression. If that's the case, you likely have a sugar-sensitivity aspect to your depression that neither you nor your doctor has recognized.

I often find myself overreacting to stress.

Volatile blood sugar levels make sugar-sensitive people edgy and reactive. You may fly off the handle or cry at the drop of a hat. The conflicting feelings you have don't seem to make sense. As an example, my client Shirley worked as a senior manager in a governmental agency. She was well thought of, did excellent work and liked her job. Most of the time she was steady and clear, but at other times she would get overwhelmed and want to sit and cry when her boss gave her feedback about her work. She was always surprised by the power of her anger, which seemed to bubble up from out of nowhere. Like Shirley, you may think of yourself as a really nice person—and most of the time you are, but at other times you feel totally out of control. These mood swings may well be due to sugar sensitivity.

I have a history of anger that sometimes surprises even me.

Sugar-sensitive people can have episodes of anger which seem to overtake them without reason. You may feel like Dr. Jekyll and Mr. Hyde. Your dark side stays hidden most of the time, but those people close to you know it's there. Your flash point is low and your impulse brakes don't work. The intensity of your feelings is particularly scary because it just doesn't seem to fit your "real" personality.

Are these patterns beginning to sound familiar? Does the sugar-sensitive profile fit your experience? Sugar-sensitive people often feel comforted by answering my diagnostic questions. Patterns which haven't made sense start fitting together.

Sugar-Sensitivity Questionnaire

In addition to answering my diagnostic questions, you can use a more formal questionnaire I have developed to determine your sugar sensitivity. Remember, though, that even this questionnaire cannot determine the exact degree of your sugar sensitivity.

Sugar sensitivity, as I am presenting it to you, is not a scientifically recognized or "proven" syndrome. It is a theory—a working hypothesis—based on my own observation of how my addicted and/or compulsive clients respond to sugars and on my in-depth investigation of the solid scientific research that has been done on carbohydrate sensitivity, and the role of brain chemicals in alcoholism, addiction and nutrition.

Five years from now your sugar sensitivity will have a scientific authority and a blood test. In the meantime, let's work with my hypothesis. The stories I have heard from my clients are too familiar and too consistent to be ignored any longer. Giving these stories a name and a solution is too important to wait for the approval of scientific authorities. I suggest you try the program I recommend as an answer to the sugar-sensitivity problem, take what fits for you and let go of the rest.

This questionnaire doesn't have a score. Its purpose is to give you information about the relationship you have to the foods that are part of the sugar-sensitive profile. The questions about whether you lied, kept a stash or went out of your way to get something sweet are included to help you look at the truth of your behavior, not to make you feel bad about it.

There's nothing bad about having a sugar-sensitive biochemistry. The more you can defuse the negative messages you have always received about your behavior, the freer you will be to begin this healing process. Remember that there are hundreds of thousands of people just like you—people who know something is wrong, who joke about being "addicted to chocolate" but rarely talk about what is really going on inside them.

As you explore the power of your own sugar sensitivity, you might want to ask yourself more questions like this. Try not to be judgmental

Sugar-Sensitivity Questionnaire

As a child, how much did you like sugar? (Rate yourself on a scale of 0—9.) ___

What kinds of sugar foods did you eat when you were a child?	How many times a day?	How many days each week?	How much did you eat each time?
Candy			
Soda			
Dessert			
Ice cream			
Straight sugar (from the bowl, cubes, honey, jelly, etc.)			
Other kinds of sweet foods (indicate which ones):			

	Yes	No
As a child, did you ever hide candy?		
As a child, did you ever steal anyone else's candy?		
As a child, did you ever steal money to buy sugar foods?		
Did you especially like the sugar and milk at the bottom of your cereal bowl?		

As an adult, how much do you like sugar? (Rate yourself on a scale of 0—9.) ___

Rate yourself for the time you were using sugar the most often as an adult.	How many times a day?	How many days each week?	How much did you eat each time?
Candy			
Soda			
Dessert			
In coffee or tea			
Ice cream/frozen yogurt			

Do you eat/drink the following? (Use the time of most frequent use as an adult.)	How many times a day?	How many days each week?	How much did you eat each time?
Fruit			
Juice			
Coffee or tea with sugar			
Alcohol			
Milk			
White breads or pastry			
Cereal			

	Yes	No
Have you ever lied about how much sweet food you ate?		
Have you ever kept a supply of sweet food on hand?		
Have you ever gotten upset if someone else ate your supply of sweet food?		
Have you ever hidden your supply from others?		
Have you ever gone out of your way to get something sweet to eat?		
Have you ever lied about how much bread you were eating?		
Have you ever hidden your supply from others?		
Have you ever gotten upset if someone else ate your supply of bread?		
Have you ever lied about how much cereal you were eating?		
Have you ever hidden your supply from others?		
Have you ever gotten upset if someone else ate your supply of cereal?		
Do you consider yourself an alcoholic?		
If so, rate the level of your alcoholism on a scale of 0–9.		
Do you ever think of sugar as "love"?		
Do you think of yourself as being addicted to sugar?		
If so, rate your sugar addiction on a scale of 0–9.		

as you do this. Allow yourself the humor of your "addiction." Perhaps you don't outright lie about when or whether you are eating sweets, but do you lie by omission? Do you eat sweets only when no one else is around? Do you put the bag with the goodies inside something else so people can't see what you are carrying? Do you park your car in an out-of-the-way place to chomp your special treat? Do you hide the candy wrappers under the other trash so your spouse won't know what you ate? Do you eat your children's cookies and then say you don't know what happened to them? Do you go to the warehouse stores and buy huge quantities of candy and tell yourself that it's a good buy? Do you know the hours of the Godiva chocolate store?

Can You Be Addicted to Sugar?

By now the answer to this question should be pretty clear to you. Yes, you can be addicted to sugar, to sweet foods and to white-flour products that your body responds to as sugars. This addiction is physiological and affects the same biochemical systems in your body as do drugs like morphine and heroin. You can actually get high on sugar. Eating it can make you feel euphoric immediately afterwards. If you don't have your regular sugar "fix," you may experience withdrawal symptoms. Yes, you can become *physiologically* dependent upon the effect the sugars have on your body.

Being sugar sensitive means you have a special biochemistry. You have a different relationship to sugar than a person with a "normal" biochemistry. Your heart sings at the sight of a newly opened box of candy, your molecules seem to jump to attention when you get a whiff of chocolate. This sensation of your body jumping to attention is not about greed. It is the natural response of a sugar-sensitive person whose brain has just released a powerful chemical called beta-endorphin in response to a certain smell.

When you eat chocolate, is there a part of you that actually feels a greater level of self-esteem? Chocolate enhancing self-esteem may seem like an outrageous idea, but chocolate releases beta-endorphin, and beta-endorphin causes an increase in feelings of self-esteem. Your relationship to sweet things is operating on a cellular level. It is much more powerful than you have realized.

In my sugar-eating past I never understood why I felt so much better after I had candy. I knew it was emotionally comforting, but it didn't make sense that I felt so good after doing something so "bad." Sometimes I would binge and start soaring with a sense of possibility about what I could do with my life. I would write plans in my journal, make lists and feel confident that the world was all right. A few hours later I would crash and feel nothing good would ever happen for me, no change would ever come, I would end up a bag lady with nothing to show for my life.

It felt crazy. How could I possibly feel such contradictory things—and feel them almost from one minute to the next? I remember the day I sat in the library working on my Ph.D. and first read about the impact of beta-endorphin on self-esteem. The hair on the back of my neck stood up. I suddenly saw the connection. I was eating chocolate as self-medication to achieve self-confidence. Instead of feeling totally stupid about my behavior, I began to see that there was wisdom in it. Consciously I wanted to feel better and more secure and unconsciously I knew there was a relationship between chocolate and self-confidence. Of course I turned to chocolate when I felt down.

The problem is, sugar-induced self-esteem doesn't last too long. And having your self-esteem wear off that quickly is a pretty fragile way to live—yes? The good news is you can evoke beta-endorphin-linked self-esteem without the negative and addictive effects of chocolate. You do not need chocolate! You need a sense of self-esteem based on an inner sense of well-being that comes from biochemical balance, clarity and well-being. What you eat can have a huge effect on how you feel. We'll see how to develop a food plan that can help you overcome the drawbacks of the sugar-sensitive body you inherited.

You can make sense of what is happening in your body. Learning about sugar sensitivity will give you a perspective that takes away the negative charge you have carried all these years about your eating. You will shift from thinking you have character defects to understanding that you have a body with a volatile blood sugar response, a low level of beta-endorphin, a low level of another brain chemical called serotonin and a heightened reaction to sweet foods. And you will learn how to change these things by what and when you eat.

The good news about biochemically based behavior is that it *can change rapidly*. You do not have to pursue years of psychotherapy to get results. You can start making sense of your patterns of behavior today to understand what foods affect you negatively and why. You can start changing what you eat and feel better right now.

As soon as you do, what has been an overwhelming—and perhaps shameful—mystery in your life will become a fascinating journey of self-exploration.

✷

Chapter 3

It's Not Your Fault

If I am right, the "crazy" duality in your life, which I call the Dr. Jekyll/Mr. Hyde syndrome, is a result of sugar sensitivity. You may *feel* crazy, but you are not. The problem is biochemical. It's not your fault.

If you are sugar sensitive, there are three things in your body chemistry that contribute to the "crazy" feelings:

- the level of sugar in your blood
- the level of the chemical serotonin in your brain
- the level of the chemical beta-endorphin in your brain

The Root of the Problem

An imbalance in the level of any *one* of these biochemicals can bring about striking changes in the way you feel or act. When all three are out of balance it is almost impossible to isolate which one is making you feel so bad. Let's take a look at them one at a time, then put them together to show you why sugar sensitivity can have such a powerful effect on your life.

You may have heard about the impact of your blood sugar level on your well-being. The effect of low serotonin levels has also been widely talked about in the last few years; books about Prozac and several "food and mood" books have examined the value of raising serotonin levels.

We'll discuss these issues—and one more. We'll look at the vital brain chemical that no one is telling the public about—beta-endorphin. And you'll see the role it plays in your feelings of self-esteem, your cravings for sugar, your capacity to handle painful situations and your feelings of hope (or despair) about the future.

As you learn about how these three biochemical systems interact to create changes in your feelings and behavior, please don't worry about the impact this information will have on the way you eat. The food plan you will develop to counteract the problem of sugar sensitivity is not about deprivation or self-denial. You'll be able to start on that plan in Chapter 6. For now, just be tender with yourself and be attentive. The story you're about to hear is intriguing.

Let's start with the most commonly known system.

The Level of Sugar in Your Blood

Your body uses a very simple form of sugar called glucose as its basic fuel. During digestion all the carbohydrates you eat are broken down into glucose. It is carried by the blood throughout your body to be

Optimal Blood Sugar	Low Blood Sugar
Energetic	Tired all the time
Tired when appropriate	Tired for no reason
Focused and relaxed	Restless, can't keep still
Clear	Confused
Having a good memory	Having trouble remembering
Able to concentrate	Having trouble concentrating
Able to solve problems effectively	Easily frustrated
Easygoing	More irritable than usual
Even-tempered	Getting angry unexpectedly

used as energy by the cells as needed. All your cells, particularly those in your brain, require a steady supply of sugar at all times.

When your body has the optimal level of sugar in the blood to supply your cells, you feel good. When your blood sugar level is too low, your cells don't get the sugar they need and they start sending out distress signals. These distress signals are the symptoms of low blood sugar, a condition known as hypoglycemia.

Brain Chemicals: Serotonin

In addition to blood sugar, a number of chemicals in your brain affect how you feel and act. Serotonin is a brain chemical that is particularly important for sugar-sensitive people. It creates a sense of relaxation, "mellows you out" and gives you a sense of being at peace with the world. Serotonin also influences your self-control, impulse control and ability to plan ahead.

Optimal Level of Serotonin	Low Level of Serotonin
Hopeful, optimistic	Depressed
Reflective and thoughtful	Impulsive
Able to concentrate	Having a short attention span
Creative, focused	Blocked, scattered
Able to think things through	Flying off the handle
Able to seek help	Suicidal
Responsive	Reactive
Looking forward to dessert without an emotional charge	Craving sweets
Hungry for a variety of different foods	Craving mostly carbohydrates like bread, pasta and cereal

When your serotonin level is low, you may feel depressed, act impulsively and have intense cravings for alcohol, sweets or carbohydrates. Scientists have worked hard to find ways to increase the level of serotonin in the brains of people who are depressed. The result is that the newer antidepressant drugs that do this—such as Prozac, Zoloft, Paxil and Effexor—have been dispensed to well over six million people.

Because of your inherited sugar sensitivity, you may find the symptoms of low serotonin familiar.

Brain Chemicals: Beta-endorphin

Beta-endorphin is the brain chemical that's gotten the least attention in the diet, depression and addiction books. That's very strange because it is immensely powerful and can drive you inexorably toward deeper addiction—or raise your spirits to a level of health that you may never have known before.

Optimal Level of Beta-endorphin	Low Level of Beta-endorphin
Having high tolerance for pain	Having low pain tolerance
Sensitive, sympathetic	Tearful, reactive
Having high self-esteem	Having low self-esteem
Compassionate	Overwhelmed by others' pain
Connected and in touch	Feeling isolated
Hopeful, optimistic, euphoric	Depressed, hopeless
Taking personal responsibility	Feeling "done to" by others
Having a take-it-or-leave-it attitude toward sweet foods	Craving sugar
Solution-oriented	Emotionally overwhelmed

When your beta-endorphin is low, you feel depressed, impulsive and victimized. You may be touchy and tearful. Your self-esteem is low. And you have a desperate craving for sugar. The scientific community has been investigating beta-endorphin for more than twenty years, but the public understanding of its effects has remained fairly limited. You may have heard of the "runner's high," a phrase that describes how the body responds to the pain of long-distance running by automatically flooding the body with beta-endorphin, which produces a sense of euphoria.

Understanding the powerful emotional effects of beta-endorphin levels in your brain is crucial for people with sugar sensitivity. The beta-endorphin story may radically change your sense of why you feel the way you do. As you see from the chart opposite, some of the effects of beta-endorphin are similar to those of serotonin.

As you've read over the symptoms on these three charts, you may have had two reactions. You may be comforted by recognizing patterns that sound so familiar and fit your experience so well. You may also be amazed that your emotional feelings and behavior can be so strongly affected by your body's chemistry.

A Delicate Balance

A normal body balances blood sugar, serotonin and beta-endorphin easily. Your sugar-sensitive body is likely off balance. The levels in all three of these systems must be optimal for you to conquer the Dr. Jekyll/Mr. Hyde syndrome. If you work on only one factor, the others will remain unbalanced. You will make some progress, but you will still experience the negative symptoms of having low levels of the other two factors.

Let's look at this visually. Here you are *before* making any change.

Low Blood Sugar	Low Level of Serotonin	Low Level of Beta-endorphin
Tired all the time	Depressed	Having low pain tolerance
Tired for no reason	Impulsive	Tearful, reactive
Restless, can't keep still	Having a short attention span	Having low self-esteem
Confused	Blocked, scattered	Overwhelmed by others' pain
Having trouble remembering	Flying off the handle	Feeling isolated
Having trouble concentrating	Suicidal	Depressed, hopeless
Easily frustrated	Reactive	Feeling "done to" by others
More irritable than usual	Craving sweets	Craving sugar!
Getting angry unexpectedly	Craving mostly carbohydrates like bread, pasta and cereal	Emotionally overwhelmed

As you can see, you feel pretty bad with all these levels out of whack. Now let's say your doctor puts you on Prozac to raise your serotonin level and ease your depression. Once you get stabilized on Prozac you start feeling better—less depressed, more optimistic and more focused. But you are still eating the way you always have—lots of sweets and starches. Let's see how things look now.

Low Blood Sugar	Optimal Level of Serotonin	Low Level of Beta-endorphin
Tired all the time	Hopeful, optimistic	Having low pain tolerance
Tired for no reason	Reflective and thoughtful	Tearful, reactive
Restless, can't keep still	Able to concentrate	Having low self-esteem
Confused	Creative, focused	Overwhelmed by others' pain
Having trouble remembering	Able to think things through	Feeling isolated
Having trouble concentrating	Able to seek help	Depressed, hopeless
Easily frustrated	Responsive	Feeling "done to" by others
More irritable than usual	Looking forward to dessert a bit	Craving sugar!
Getting angry unexpectedly	Hungry for healthy foods	Emotionally overwhelmed

So although your depression is lifting, your self-esteem is still low and you feel isolated and emotionally overwhelmed. How can you explain this? It doesn't make any sense. The Prozac is supposed to help—and it does. But why do the black feelings still come? They aren't as bad as in the past, but something is still off. And you are still exhausted at five in the afternoon.

Here is what is happening. You have raised your serotonin level, but your blood sugar and beta-endorphin levels remain low. You still get tired and feel crabby, and your self-esteem wobbles a lot. You feel isolated and overwhelmed and find it hard to concentrate. Your first thought may be that your medication isn't working. You may shift to another drug like Paxil or Zoloft, and for a while things improve. Then the same problems come back. But you are committed to feeling better, so you keep searching for solutions.

Perhaps you come across one of the popular diet books like *Dr. Atkins' New Diet Revolution* or Barry Sears's *Mastering the Zone* that talk about needing to stabilize your blood sugar by eating more protein or "balancing" each of your meals with a specific ratio of protein, fat and carbohydrate. These dietary plans identify many of the symptoms you feel. So you decide to drop the medication altogether and start one of these diets. It stabilizes your blood sugar and you begin to feel better.

Here's what that looks like:

Optimal Blood Sugar	Low Level of Serotonin	Low Level of Beta-endorphin
Energetic	Depressed	Having low pain tolerance
Tired when appropriate	Impulsive	Tearful, reactive
Focused and relaxed	Having a short attention span	Having low self-esteem
Clear	Blocked, scattered	Overwhelmed by others' pain
Having a good memory	Flying off the handle	Feeling isolated
Able to concentrate	Suicidal	Depressed, hopeless
Able to solve problems effectively	Reactive	Feeling "done to" by others
Easygoing	Craving sweets	Craving sugar!
Even-tempered	Craving mostly carbohydrates like bread, pasta and cereal	Emotionally overwhelmed

Once again, you start to feel better. But trouble is coming. As it turns out, the very behaviors that make these diets improve your blood sugar level will decrease your level of serotonin and make your low-serotonin symptoms worse. And if you use sweets to create the carbohydrate balance advocated in *Mastering the Zone*, you will also make your low beta-endorphin symptoms worse.

One problem is that many of these new diets advocate the use of "specially balanced" nutrition bars. These bars are advertised as low-fat, natural and healthy. But they often contain high levels of what

their labels call carbohydrates, which are actually sugars that will
activate your low-beta-endorphin symptoms. Chapter 5 will tell you
all about how this happens. These nutrition bars are very compelling
for sugar-sensitive people. You may find yourself wanting to eat several
bars a day. But thanks to your inherited sugar sensitivity, what starts
off as convenience becomes dependence.

However, you are on the right track in wanting to stabilize your
blood sugar. If you forgo nutrition bars that are made with sugars, stop
using sugars and white-flour products (which your body reacts to like
sugar), and eat complex carbohydrates (like beans or whole grains) to
achieve the diet's balancing process, you can avoid the problem with
your beta-endorphin.

Now things are getting better. You have improved two of the
factors creating your Dr. Jekyll/Mr. Hyde syndrome. Take a look at
the next chart.

Optimal Blood Sugar	Low Level of Serotonin	Optimal Level of Beta-endorphin
Energetic	Depressed	Having high tolerance for pain
Tired when appropriate	Impulsive	Sensitive, sympathetic
Focused and relaxed	Having a short attention span	Having high self-esteem
Clear	Blocked, scattered	Compassionate
Having a good memory	Flying off the handle	Connected and in touch
Able to concentrate	Suicidal	Hopeful, optimistic, euphoric
Able to solve problems effectively	Reactive	Taking personal responsibility
Easygoing	Craving sweets	Having a take-it-or-leave-it attitude toward sweet foods
Even-tempered	Craving mostly carbohydrates like bread, pasta and cereal	Solution-oriented

As you can see, this is a huge improvement. You have balanced
your blood sugar and your beta-endorphin. However, you still have a
problem. Within a few weeks you will begin to feel desperate. Your

depression will return with a vengeance and you will feel completely discouraged because you are doing all the right things and you still feel bad.

This is why balancing the levels of all three of these important biochemicals is so crucial to your well-being as a sugar-sensitive person. And you can do it with simple food and lifestyle changes. On the next chart you'll see the profile that can be yours by using the nutritional approach I have developed for people with inherited sugar sensitivity.

Optimal Blood Sugar	Optimal Level of Serotonin	Optimal Level of Beta-endorphin
Energetic	Hopeful, optimistic	Having high tolerance for pain
Tired when appropriate	Reflective and thoughtful	Sensitive, sympathetic
Focused and relaxed	Able to concentrate	Having high self-esteem
Clear	Creative, focused	Compassionate
Having a good memory	Able to think things through	Connected and in touch
Able to concentrate	Able to seek help	Hopeful, optimistic, euphoric
Able to solve problems effectively	Responsive	Taking personal responsibility
Easygoing	Looking forward to dessert a bit	Having a take-it-or-leave-it attitude toward sweet foods
Even-tempered	Hungry for healthy foods	Solution-oriented

You don't have to settle for one or two out of three. You can have optimal levels in all these vital systems.

The healing process I have developed will allow you to design your own food plan, one that will specifically target your needs and personal priorities. Using it, you will learn to read your own body to see which factor is contributing to your symptoms. You will learn which foods contribute to your overall health and when it is best for you to eat them. As you will discover in Chapter 7, when you eat is almost as important as what you eat.

Learning this process won't happen overnight. There is no magic pill that makes everything work all at once. You will have to put effort into it. But the process is very simple and you will start feeling better rapidly. As you come to understand how your blood sugar, serotonin and beta-endorphin levels affect you, you will become more and more excited about the mastery you can achieve. The Dr. Jekyll/ Mr. Hyde syndrome is not a life sentence!

✪

Chapter 4

The Ups and Downs of Blood Sugar

Because you are sugar sensitive, you respond differently to sugar than other people do. This is most immediately apparent in the effect of what you eat on your blood sugar level. People with normal body chemistries can eat sweet foods without experiencing dramatic changes in their blood sugar level, but for you the story is different. When you eat something sweet, the result is not the pleasant spurt of energy caused by a slight *increase* in your blood sugar level, but all the devastating feelings brought on by a sharp *decrease* in blood sugar. Let's take a closer look.

How Normal Blood Sugar Works

The level of sugar in your blood fluctuates with eating, sleeping and other activities. When you eat, your blood sugar level goes up. When you use energy, your blood sugar level goes down. The most important thing for you to understand about your blood sugar level is that because you are sugar sensitive, it has a very powerful effect on how you feel. If your brain or your muscles can't get the blood sugar they need to perform, they will tell you very clearly that something is wrong. You may get tired, shaky or irritable. You may have a hard time concentrating. You may forget things. You may reach for something sweet to provide a quick pick-me-up.

Most of the sugar in your blood comes from the foods you eat. The rest comes from the extra sugar stored in your liver, which is to be used if you run out of food for energy. The most efficient source of sugar for the average person is carbohydrates because they require the least amount of work by the body to convert them from "food" to sugar in your blood. Carbohydrates can either be simple, like beer, sugar and white flour, or they can be complex, like potatoes, oatmeal and whole grains. The simpler a carbohydrate is, the more quickly it can be broken down into glucose (the simplest sugar) and released into your bloodstream, where it can be carried to your cells and burned for energy. The more complex a carbohydrate is, the longer it takes to be broken down and released into the blood.

Your body's goal is to maintain the perfect level of sugar in your blood—neither too high nor too low. Your body uses a number of mechanisms to achieve this. First, it draws from the regular sugar pool in your blood. Your body does this by releasing a hormone called insulin, which instructs your cells to open up, move sugar out of your blood and pull it into the cells themselves, where it can be burned for fuel. When the level of sugar in your blood goes up, your body releases more insulin and thereby moves more sugar into your cells. This not only provides fuel for your cells, it also keeps your blood sugar level on an even keel.

If the level of sugar in your blood drops, your body will turn to the backup sugar supply stored in your liver. Your liver stores about 400 calories worth of sugar at any given time. After this backup supply is used up, you are in trouble. Your body needs more sugar to keep functioning. It tells you to eat. Now!

For most people, this system works well. They are not even aware of the changes in their blood sugar level. However, some people are biochemically sugar sensitive. When they eat sugar, their bodies overreact by releasing far more insulin than is needed. The result is that their cells open up and pull in more sugar than they should. This causes the level of sugar in the blood to drop too low and triggers those "crazy" Mr. Hyde symptoms of low blood sugar, including fatigue, restlessness, confusion, frustration, poor memory and irritability.

The Impact of Sugar Sensitivity

Sugar-sensitive people have a more volatile blood sugar reaction to eating sweet foods than do other people. If you are sugar sensitive, your blood sugar rises more quickly and goes higher than other people's, causing your body to release more insulin than is needed for the amount of food you have eaten. As a result of this spike in insulin, you experience a quicker and steeper drop in your blood sugar level. You are more vulnerable to low blood sugar level, also known as hypoglycemia.

Let's look at the blood sugar response of a person who is not sugar sensitive. Mary is a "normal," active working woman. She gets up, has a breakfast of oatmeal, whole grain toast, juice and one cup of coffee with sweetener around seven in the morning. She has a turkey sandwich, chips and a glass of milk for lunch at around one in the afternoon, drinks a cup of tea when she gets home from work, then eats a piece of chicken, a baked potato and green beans for dinner at about six-thirty in the evening. She has a piece of apple pie for dessert.

This is what Mary's blood sugar curve might look like:

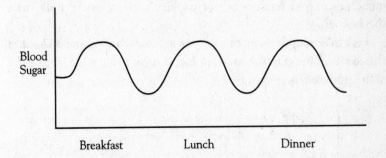

Mary's blood sugar is low when she gets up because she hasn't eaten since the night before. Her sugar level rises after breakfast and then begins to fall as her body uses the sugar for energy. The drop in her blood sugar around noon signals her body that it's time to eat. Mary recognizes these signals and has lunch. Her sugar level rises as her body digests the food she has eaten. As the sugar in that food is used for energy, her blood sugar level will begin to drop in the afternoon. When Mary eats dinner, her blood sugar rises again. After dinner and while she sleeps, her sugar level eventually drops back to where it started at the beginning of the day. Overall, her blood sugar level is pretty stable and predictable. There are no extreme peaks or valleys.

Let's look at what your blood sugar curve—as a sugar-sensitive person—might be. Your typical day might start like this. You get up at seven and grab a cup of coffee with 2 teaspoons of sugar and some cream before you race out the door. You stop on the way to work and pick up a second cup of coffee (with the same cream and sugar) and a chocolate muffin. At ten you have another cup of coffee with 2 teaspoons of sugar and more cream. You are so busy working that you forget to eat lunch. At three in the afternoon you get really tired and feel as if you are going to fall off the cliff, so you go to the deli downstairs and get a pasta salad and some iced tea. At four-thirty you are really sleepy so you get a Coke from the machine. You get home at seven, pour yourself a glass of wine to unwind and watch the news. You go poke around the refrigerator for something to eat. Finding nothing, you boil water, cook some pasta, put butter and cheese on it, and eat it while watching TV. At nine you get the munchies so you fetch a bag of cookies and a glass of milk from the kitchen.

Let's take your day a piece at a time and see what's going on behind the scenes. This graph shows your blood sugar rising after having the coffee and muffin.

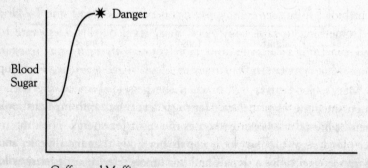

As you now know, sugar-sensitive people overreact to eating simple carbohydrates; blood sugar goes up higher and more quickly than other people's. The sugar in your coffee and the chocolate muffin created a blood sugar spike and your body gets the message that something is wrong. It registers DANGER! and goes into action to get the extra sugar out of your blood. Your body wants to maintain the correct level of sugar within your blood. If there is too much, your pancreas will release insulin to move the sugar from your blood into your cells. If your blood sugar spikes up, your body will tell your pancreas to release a big hit of insulin, which instructs your cells to open up and use the sugar. This rush of insulin does its job, and you experience a rapid and steep drop in your blood sugar level.

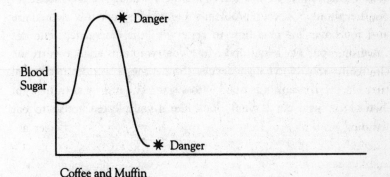

Because of this big hit of insulin, your blood sugar drops dramatically, and your body *again* registers DANGER! and gets mobilized to find a solution. This time the danger comes from having too little sugar in your blood. Whether consciously or unconsciously, you start looking for something to raise your blood sugar level quickly. Desperate to find something sweet, you drink more coffee with sugar in it. You can guess what happens now with your blood sugar level. It shoots up again.

If you chart these ups and downs during the day, they might look the graph on the following page.

You can see that your body experiences these dramatic peaks and valleys several times a day. What are the consequences of these wild fluctuations in your blood sugar levels? The first is simple. Your moods,

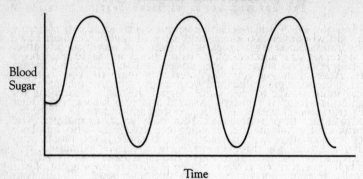

like your blood sugar, fluctuate all day. Sometimes you feel high and sometimes you feel low. You may feel focused and alert for 30 minutes after eating, but then you can't remember whom you are talking to on the phone. Or your problem-solving skills suddenly desert you and you haven't a clue how to cope with the emergency that just came up. Your Dr. Jekyll and Mr. Hyde symptoms change with the change in your blood sugar levels. (Sometimes I wonder if the vial that Dr. Jekyll drank was filled with sugar.) What do you think your own blood sugar curve would look like if you plotted it throughout the day?

Adrenal Fatigue

In addition, each time your blood sugar spikes so quickly, your body's internal alarms start ringing and signal your adrenal glands to release adrenaline, the hormone that gives you a quick surge of energy and mobilizes you in the face of danger. This response kept our ancestors alive when they were being chased by saber-toothed tigers. You can feel that zing today when you have a near-miss accident while driving to work or when someone comes up from behind and takes you by surprise. The adrenaline rush makes your heart pump faster and makes you more alert. (It also tells your pancreas to get in gear and release insulin to reduce the high level of sugar in your blood.)

The problem is, your adrenal glands are designed for coping with emergencies. They are not built to go into action several times a day, as they do whenever you eat a large dose of sugar. So when blood sugar spikes set your adrenals off morning, noon and night, they begin to tire. Adrenal fatigue sets in. When that happens, your adrenals respond more slowly to the danger signal. Instead of catching the rapidly rising blood sugar early, they go into action late.

Think of the adrenals as a volunteer firefighter who has been working overtime for three months. He is totally exhausted. The alarm bell rings at three in the morning. Instead of leaping out of bed, he vaguely hears the alarm, struggles to focus, finally recognizes that it is the bell ringing rather than his dream, stumbles out of bed, gropes for his boots, walks to his truck, slumps at the wheel, then finally gets mobilized to turn the motor on and get to the fire. He used to leap from his bed, drop his feet into his boots in an instant and be out the door before the bell had finished ringing. But his fatigue is clobbering his response time.

Because your adrenals are reacting late, your blood sugar has risen even higher and your body releases even more insulin in an attempt to get that sugar out of your blood and into your cells. The result is that the peaks and valleys in your blood sugar level get steeper and the interval between them gets shorter. Your blood sugar curve starts to look like this:

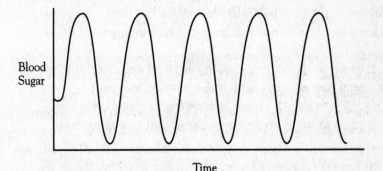

Blood
Sugar

Time

Ironically, adrenal fatigue—which is caused by your body's over-reaction to sugar—means you need more sugar more often because you drop into the lower danger zone more and more frequently. Thus adrenal fatigue makes your blood sugar ups and downs even *more* pronounced and some of your Mr. Hyde symptoms may get even worse. You may not be aware that this change for the worse is related to what you eat and when you eat it. You may think your bad feelings are caused by stress, lack of sleep or PMS. Think about how often you experience the following symptoms:

❏ Fatigue	❏ Irritability
❏ Restlessness	❏ Difficulty remembering
❏ Confusion	❏ Anger (men)
❏ Shakiness	❏ Feeling weepy (women)
❏ Frustration	❏ Anxiety

It's no wonder you don't feel well. You are riding a physiological roller coaster. Because you are sugar sensitive and because of what and when you eat, your blood sugar can't be counted on to remain stable and give you a reliable and steady source of energy. By three in the afternoon, you feel as if you are crawling through the day. By seven, you can hardly get it together to make dinner.

But the problem is not in your mind. It is not a matter of attitude. Unless you stabilize your blood sugar, no amount of counseling or insight will help you feel better. That's the bad news. The good news is that you can solve this problem by understanding three things:

1. which foods will give you a stable blood sugar level that will not send your adrenal glands into action unnecessarily
2. which foods will evoke the least reactive insulin response
3. when to eat to keep your energy up and your spirits high

In the next chapter we'll look at the two other key players in defeating your body's sugar sensitivity, the brain chemicals serotonin and beta-endorphin. Then you'll start putting into action a food plan that can give you the emotional stability and high self-esteem you've wanted—and deserved—for so long.

Chapter 5

✪

Brain Chemistry 101

While extreme highs and lows in your blood sugar level can have a devastating effect on how you feel, getting your blood sugar stable will not solve all the problems of the Dr. Jekyll/Mr. Hyde syndrome. If it could, you would not need to read this book. A number of experts have written on the importance of blood sugar levels to emotional well-being.

But there's more to our sugar-sensitivity story, and it includes some crucial information that has not been widely available to the public before. This information is about the crucial importance of beta-endorphin, one of the two brain chemicals we discussed briefly at the beginning of Chapter 3. Beta-endorphin and its better-known partner, serotonin, can have dramatically positive—or negative—effects on your moods and your energy level.

The way these brain chemicals work is a little more complex than the mechanics of blood sugar, and you will need some background in how the brain works. If you'd rather skip the details about the science and get started on your food plan, turn to Chapter 6. As you design your plan, you'll find out which of its seven steps will affect your blood sugar, serotonin and beta-endorphin levels. That way you can return to the material in this section as you reach each step.

In the long run, however, taking the time to learn about how your brain works will provide you with a real sense of confidence. It will help you to understand the subtle nuances of what you are feeling and the reasons you are feeling it. You can learn the difference between feelings based on blood sugar fluctuations, serotonin levels and beta-endorphin levels. This ability to identify the specific physiological changes behind your feelings and behavior becomes incredibly exciting. The skill puts you in the driver's seat and gives you a way to chart your life as you never have before. As I have seen time and again in my clients, this exhilarating feeling of self-confidence is well worth the effort to understand the material.

We'll begin this chapter by taking a look at neurotransmitters, the family of brain chemicals to which serotonin and beta-endorphin belong. As we saw in Chapter 3, they have a powerful effect on your moods and behavior. You'll learn the purpose of neurotransmitters, the mechanism by which they send information between brain cells and what the brain does to try to keep this information flow steady. Then we'll look specifically at serotonin and beta-endorphin and examine how traditional drugs, both prescription and nonprescription, affect the neurotransmitters. Finally, we'll see why and how using food can provide an ideal alternative for balancing your brain chemistry.

Neurotransmitters: Messengers of the Brain

Your brain is designed to communicate information. Billions of brain cells talk to each other moment by moment through a complex network of interconnecting cells. These cells do not actually touch one another. There is a tiny space between each of them and information is passed across this space by way of chemical messengers called neurotransmitters.

There are many kinds of neurotransmitters, each of which has a different molecular shape and carries its own distinct message. When one brain cell wants to send a message to another, it releases the appropriate type of neurotransmitter into the space between it and the receiving cell. These neurotransmitters float across this tiny space and look for a place to land. Each receiving cell has thousands of receptors ready to catch its neurotransmitters. These are called neuro-receptors and each is designed to match a neurotransmitter.

A molecule of serotonin, for example, can only pass its message to a serotonin receptor. The same is true with beta-endorphin. If any other kind of neurotransmitter hits the beta-endorphin receptors, nothing happens. But when the neurotransmitter that fits the receptor comes along, the receptor recognizes it and allows the message to pass. If enough receptors get the same message, then the entire cell responds and passes the message to the next cell. Of course, this all happens in a very, very short time. Let's look at how this communication works with our two neurotransmitters, beta-endorphin and serotonin.

First, here's an example of how beta-endorphin, which eases physical and emotional pain, works. Mary drops a heavy box on her fingers. Her first response is one of intense pain. She is nauseous and feels as if she will pass out. However, before too long, she feels clear and focused. Her fingers still hurt, but she knows that ice will reduce the swelling and help to numb the pain.

While Mary is standing at the sink with her fingers in a bowl of ice water, she is surprised to notice that she feels a little relaxed and spacey. This seems strange since she just smashed her fingers. But Mary's brain recognized a crisis when the pain sensations started to reach it and responded by releasing beta-endorphin molecules that blunted those throbbing sensations.

Let's take an even closer look at this painkilling mechanism. Mary's beta-endorphin molecules are stored in her brain cells. When the sending cells recognized pain, they released beta-endorphin. The beta-endorphin molecules crossed the space between brain cells and hit the beta-endorphin receptors on the receiving cells, causing the cell to receive the message and respond to it. Because Mary felt much pain, a lot of beta-endorphin was released and a powerful pain-blocking message got through.

Second, let's see how serotonin, which deals with mood and behavior, functions. Diane is sugar sensitive. She is also a compulsive eater who loves certain foods. She often talks about wanting to lose weight, but when she goes out to a restaurant one evening and bread appears on the table while she is waiting for her dinner to be served, her resolve evaporates. Diane has low levels of serotonin, the neurotransmitter which puts the brakes on impulses. Because she is sugar sensitive, Diane's behavior "brakes" don't always work.

If Diane had the body chemistry of a normal person, her brain would have an adequate level of serotonin, which would enable her to recognize the message to "eat bread now" as impulsive behavior (as opposed to actual hunger) and not act on it. But because Diane's serotonin levels are naturally low, there is less flowing between her brain cells. This small amount of serotonin crosses the space between her brain cells, finds the serotonin receptors and passes along the message to stop, which should defuse Diane's impulse to eat. But because there isn't very much serotonin, the message remains pretty weak. Not enough of the receptors are activated, so the cells don't pass the message along, and Diane's impulse to eat the bread is not quieted. Instead, she practically inhales the bread, eating way more than she really wants to.

Let's imagine that we can increase Diane's serotonin levels. She still feels bad about her eating patterns and still looks at the bread on her table, thinking, I will just have a little of this bread while I am waiting. But before she pops a piece into her mouth, something happens. A little voice says, Wait a minute, Diane. Are you sure that's the best thing to do? So Diane thinks about it a little. She sighs and thinks, Well, um, maybe that's not such a good idea. Diane has just exercised impulse control, courtesy of serotonin.

When we increased Diane's imaginary serotonin level, there were many more serotonin molecules hitting the receptors, and the cells passed the message throughout her brain, in effect telling her to wait. Diane's impulse quieted down as the message got through. She got another benefit from increasing her level of serotonin: her feelings of irritability, isolation and depression were quieted as well. Diane didn't understand how all this worked in her brain. She didn't have a clue about the serotonin action. And she didn't need to. She just felt more in control of her life and her behavior. Diane's brain knew exactly what it was doing, though: more serotonin equals impulse control and better feelings. Later, you'll learn how to increase your serotonin (and your beta-endorphin) by changing the foods you eat and doing other things like exercising, meditating or praying, laughing and even having good sex!

Cleaning Up and Regulating the System

After a neurotransmitter hits its receptor and passes its message along, it floats back into the space between brain cells and is available to hit the receptors again. At the same time, the sending cell keeps releasing more of the same neurotransmitter, creating a risk of overload. To prevent this, your brain has a couple of ways to get rid of the "leftover" serotonin or beta-endorphin molecules. First, it releases enzymes that break down the used neurotransmitters. I like to think of each enzyme as a little Pac-Man chomping the used neurotransmitters. The other mechanism that prevents neurotransmitter overload is a sort of vacuum cleaner that sucks up the used messengers and deposits them back in the sending cell to be recycled for later use. These "vacuum cleaners," called reuptake pumps, are, like the Pac-Man enzymes, usually very effective in doing this cleanup. Your brain not only wants things cleaned up, it also wants them orderly and organized. That's why the brain's system of neurotransmitters and neuroreceptors is carefully orchestrated to stay in balance. If things get unbalanced, your brain will try to compensate for the problem.

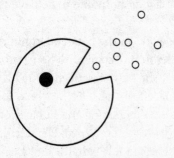

Pac-Man Eating Used Neurotransmitters

Three of these adjustments are particularly important for our story. These are downregulation, upregulation and withdrawal.

Downregulation

Receiving too much of any given message confuses your brain. It doesn't like being overloaded. If too much serotonin or beta-endorphin is released, the receiving cell will close down some of its receptors, thereby limiting the number of hits it can receive. Even though there are more neurotransmitters released, there are fewer places for them to land. This process of closing down receptors is called downregulation.

Downregulation is what causes people to develop a tolerance to a drug. Let's use painkilling drugs as an example. Painkillers like morphine work because their molecules are shaped like beta-endorphin molecules. They fit into the beta-endorphin receptors and pass along the painkilling message. But when you take a painkilling drug, you get many more hits than you would normally. So your brain, which values balance above all else, wants to get things back to normal. After a while it closes down some of its receptors. In other words, it downregulates. Downregulation means your brain cells are getting fewer hits, so the same amount of your painkiller has less effect. This is what has happened when you develop a tolerance for a drug and need a bigger dose to do the job. Downregulation happens fairly quickly. You might need 50 mg of morphine to get relief from pain on the first day and 500 mg of morphine to achieve the same effect ten days later.

Just as painkillers work on the beta-endorphin system, antidepressants work on the serotonin system. When Barbara started taking Prozac for depression, she was prescribed 20 mg a day. After getting over some initial side effects, she felt a whole lot better for a few months. The Prozac was increasing the number of serotonin hits in her brain. Then her depression returned. Her doctor upped the dosage to 40 mg a day and Barbara felt better again. But over time the bad feelings started creeping back in. Barbara's brain was downregulating in response to the increase in the serotonin hits, so the Prozac now had less of an effect. Here's a picture to show you how downregulation works:

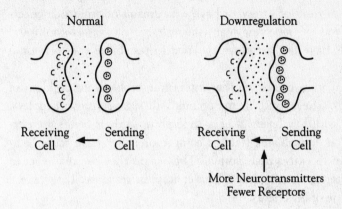

Upregulation

The brain-chemistry balancing system works in the other direction as well. If your level of serotonin or beta-endorphin gets too low, your brain will open up more receptors so it can get more hits. Here is a picture that shows upregulation:

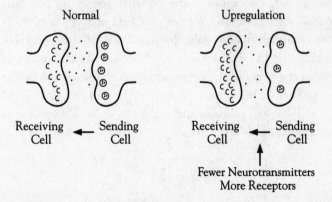

Upregulation creates some interesting problems. If you are sugar sensitive and have naturally low levels of serotonin, then you also have more serotonin receptors. This means that if you start taking a drug like Prozac, you may have a very big reaction to it. All of a sudden you are getting more serotonin hits in a system that was already upregulated to have many extra serotonin receptors. So you may feel anxious or jittery, or have wild dreams or other side effects because you are receiving many, many more hits of serotonin and your cells have not yet downregulated to restabilize your serotonin level.

Upregulation causes another interesting problem for children of alcoholics. They—and, in my opinion, all sugar-sensitive people— are born with low levels of beta-endorphin, so their brains are normally in an upregulated state to compensate: they have more beta-endorphin receptors than normal. This means they can overreact to any substance that evokes a beta-endorphin response. Let's take a look at one of my clients.

Joe, a twelve-year-old son of an alcoholic, has low levels of beta-endorphin. On the outside he acts cool when hanging out with his buddies, but inside he doesn't feel too good about himself. One day Joe and his buddies sneak a six-pack of beer. His buddies have normal brain chemistry. They drink a can or two of beer and feel good, slightly high and pretty relaxed.

But Joe's brain has far more endorphin receptors because his own natural level of beta-endorphin is low. So when Joe drinks two cans of beer, POW! Alcohol causes a release of beta-endorphin with its capacity for easing emotional pain. Joe is on top of the world. He feels better than he has in his whole life because his extra receptors have amplified the effect of the beta-endorphin release caused by the alcohol in the beer. "This is great," Joe says. And will he drink again? You bet he will. He will probably spend the rest of his life seeking to relive the euphoria of his first drink.

Withdrawal

The third way your brain tries to recover from imbalance is by creating withdrawal symptoms. When you develop a physical dependence on a substance—such as a morphine-based painkiller, alcohol or sugar—you have altered the natural state of your system. Your brain gets used to having the extra serotonin or beta-endorphin hits caused by the substance and it "complains" if the substance is cut off. You experience these complaints as withdrawal symptoms such as irritability, headaches, diarrhea, joint pains and other flulike symptoms.

When you are experiencing withdrawal and you take the substance your neuroreceptors are screaming for, you immediately feel better—at least for a little while. This rapid improvement is one of the best ways to test whether the feelings you are experiencing come from physical withdrawal. If you immediately feel better when you give your body what it craves, it's a strong clue that you are dealing with physical dependency and withdrawal.

Now that you have a better sense of the overall chemistry affecting your brain process, let's take a deeper look at the specific neurotransmitters affecting the sugar-sensitive person.

Serotonin

As we saw in Chapter 3, when your serotonin level is in an ideal state you feel mellow and relaxed. You have a sense of being at peace with life. Serotonin also increases impulse control, which allows you to more easily "just say no." People with low levels of serotonin do not have good impulse control. It is almost impossible for them to "just say no" because there is such a short time period between the urge to do something and doing it. This is why the warm cookies on the kitchen table hop into your mouth before you even know what has happened. This is why no matter how many times you vow to stick with your diet, you are not able to. The insufficient serotonin level in your brain isn't giving you the time you need to make good decisions.

Besides being impulsive, people with low levels of serotonin can feel depressed and often find themselves craving simple carbohydrates such as bread, pasta or candy. When your brain is low in serotonin, it works to do whatever it can to increase it. Not only does it upregulate, or open up more receptors to grab whatever serotonin your brain cells are releasing, it also produces cravings for foods that will raise your serotonin level. Simple carbohydrates do this. Here's how.

Serotonin is made from the chemical tryptophan, an amino acid that comes from protein. But while eating turkey will get tryptophan into your blood, this won't necessarily mean that the tryptophan will actually get into your brain to make serotonin. You need simple carbohydrates to move the tryptophan into your brain, where it can be used to make serotonin. We'll talk more about how to use tryptophan to raise your spirits, improve your sleep and help you feel more relaxed in Chapter 7, but for now remember that snacking on a carbohydrate can raise the level of serotonin in your brain *if you've eaten enough protein first* to get tryptophan into your bloodstream.

This fact has encouraged a number of authors to recommend eating sweets—in particular chocolate—as the ideal alternative to antidepressant drugs. I strongly disagree. While chocolate does raise serotonin levels, it is not the best solution for raising your serotonin levels *and* relieving depression. Chocolate may work for someone else, but not for you. You are sugar sensitive. When you eat chocolate you will get a rise in your serotonin level, but at a huge price. Chocolate will backfire on you by increasing your craving for sweets and reinforcing your addiction. You'll see why this happens in the section on beta-endorphin.

How Antidepressants Work

Another school of thought says that the best way to raise low serotonin levels—and thereby relieve depression—is to take an antidepressant drug. Most antidepressants work by increasing the number of serotonin molecules received by the neuroreceptors. The scientists who developed antidepressants focused on creating drugs that would cause the original low number of serotonin molecules released by a depressed person's brain cells to remain in the space between cells for a longer time, thus allowing these molecules to hit the serotonin receptors more than once. Some antidepressants do this by blocking the Pac-Man enzyme that gobbles up secondhand serotonin; others work by stopping the reuptake pumps from vacuuming up the used neurotransmitters.

Drugs like Prozac, Paxil, Effexor and Zoloft belong to the second type. They turn off the reuptake pumps so secondhand serotonin stays between cells and continues to hit the serotonin receptors. In effect, your brain is getting more use out of the serotonin you have. These antidepressants tend to work better than the Pac-Man-blocking kind because they have fewer side effects.

The good thing about drugs like Prozac is that they do increase your serotonin level and improve the problem moods and behaviors associated with low serotonin. As we saw in Chapter 3, higher levels of serotonin make you less depressed, less scattered, more focused, less blocked, less irritable and less likely to crave sweets, bread, pasta or cereal. Thanks to improved impulse control, you are also better able to say no to alcohol, food and compulsive behaviors.

As with the chocolate "solution," however, there are significant problems with taking antidepressants. First, as we saw in Barbara's case, your brain will close down some receptors after a while in response to the increase in serotonin caused by the antidepressant and you will have to increase your dose or change the type of medication you are using to get the same effect. Second, many of these drugs are very expensive and must be taken under the supervision of a psychiatrist, and your treatment may not be covered by your health insurance. And third, even these newer antidepressants have unpleasant side effects. You may experience nausea, jitteriness, weird dreams or problems with your sleep. You may find that you have no sexual drive, are less sensitive physically to sexual stimulation and cannot achieve orgasm. While antidepressants can be lifesaving if you have a serious depression that does not respond to anything else, the side effects may be a high price to pay for this relief.

There are other options. Certain ways of eating can significantly alter your serotonin levels. What and when you eat can be a wonderful ally in your seven-step process. If you eat a baked potato (with the skin) as a snack before bed, you will put the biochemistry in motion to get the tryptophan into your brain to make serotonin. As you continue to read this book, you will begin to see why potatoes may be a better alternative than Prozac.

Beta-endorphin

Let's turn to the other neurotransmitter important for sugar-sensitive people, beta-endorphin. Beta-endorphin acts as a powerful natural painkiller. We've discussed the runner's high (also called an endorphin rush), whereby the body responds to the pain of long-distance running by flooding the brain with beta-endorphin. Your natural beta-endorphin is incredibly potent and serves you well. The problem for sugar-sensitive people, however, is that their "normal" level of beta-endorphin may be low and their natural response to a beta-endorphin releasing substance (like sugar) may be significantly greater than that of people with ordinary body chemistry. As we'll see later, that can cause huge problems.

In scientific terms, beta-endorphin is an endogenous opioid, meaning that it can be found naturally in the body and that it has an opiumlike effect, as heroin and morphine do. Like the other opioids, proper levels of beta-endorphin produce a sense of well-being, reduce pain, ease emotional distress, increase self-esteem, create affective stability and even create a sense of euphoria. Not surprisingly, beta-endorphin also controls anxiety, defuses paranoid feelings, reduces anger and relieves certain types of depression. With all these positive effects coming from sufficient beta-endorphin, you can see the problems you run into when your system isn't producing enough. If your beta-endorphin level is naturally low, you will have to live with low self-esteem that is *biochemically* based and is not responsive to psychotherapy or counseling.

Narcotics such as morphine, heroin and codeine work like beta-endorphin because their molecules have the same shape. They can fit into the beta-endorphin receptor sites and fool the brain into thinking that more natural beta-endorphin was sent. The result is the same as that produced by our own beta-endorphin: high tolerance to pain, a sense of euphoria, optimism and high self-esteem.

As we saw in the case of Joe, alcohol also has a beta-endorphin effect on the brain. It does not act on the receptors directly, as narcotics do, but causes the brain to release additional beta-endorphin to produce the high we associate with drinking. And since we sugar-sensitive people have naturally lower levels of beta-endorphins, our brains have opened up more receptors to receive what's there—and we get an even bigger high from drinking than many of our buddies. Like Joe, we tend to really like the effect alcohol produces. Sugar-sensitive people have a greater reaction to all the things that evoke a beta-endorphin response, as we will see.

Sugar and the Beta-endorphin Response

Let's go back to our old friend sugar in the context of this heightened beta-endorphin response. Like alcohol, sugar causes a release of beta-endorphin. It can make you feel high and reduce both physical and emotional pain. Normal people can enjoy this property of sugar without ill effects. But sugar-sensitive people respond to the beta-endorphin effect of sugar in a bigger way because they naturally have so many more receptors. For them, eating sugar can be like drinking alcohol! Sugar can make us funny, relaxed, silly, talkative and temporarily self-confident.

If you are sugar sensitive, you have no doubt experienced this druglike effect after eating sugar. Unfortunately, this response is not usually taken seriously. People make jokes about being a "choco-holic," but rarely speak of the real pain caused by the continuing and compulsive use of sweets.

A number of scientists and physicians have been interested in how sugar affects our minds and bodies. In fact, people have been writing about the harmful effects of sugar since the early 1950s. But most of these publications weren't taken seriously by the medical community. They tended to be dismissed as "unscientific" and "anecdotal."

But more recently, scientists have started looking at sugars in a more focused way. In the mid-1980s, Dr. Elliott Blass, now a researcher at Cornell University, conducted some fascinating experiments that looked at the possibility of using sugar as a safe analgesic (painkiller) for babies. To test his hypothesis that sugar could be used in this way, Blass timed the reactions of a group of mice exposed to a potentially painful level of heat. He first rested the front foot of a mouse on a hot plate and then measured how quickly it lifted its paw from the heat. The mice lifted their little feet up in an average of 10 seconds.

Blass then gave the mice a drink that was 11.5 percent sugar and repeated the experiment. This time it took them an average of 20 seconds—twice as long—to lift those little paws. These results suggested that the sugar was blocking the pain of the heat; it was acting like a painkiller.

Blass then tried to establish the neurochemical basis for what he was seeing. He had observed that the ingestion of sugar was reducing the mice's pain response, but he wasn't sure which neurochemical pathway was involved. It was Blass's belief that the sugar somehow acted like an opioid—perhaps by causing a release of the natural painkiller beta-endorphin—so he designed an experiment using the drug Naltrexone to test his hypothesis. Naltrexone, which blocks the painkilling effect of opioid drugs such as morphine and heroin, works by sitting in the beta-endorphin receptors and preventing them from receiving the soothing, painkilling message that beta-endorphin wants to transmit to the body. Blass reasoned that if Naltrexone also blocked the painkilling effect of sugar (which he would learn by observing whether the mice reacted quickly or not to the hot plate), it would mean that sugar acted on the brain—and specifically the beta-endorphin system—like an opioid.

In his new experiment, Blass gave the mice a dose of Naltrexone before giving them the sugar drink. Then he tested their reaction to the hot plate. The mice picked up their little feet real quickly. This time those little paws were up in 8 seconds as if they were saying, "That thing is HOT!!!" The Naltrexone had indeed blocked the painkilling effect of the sugar. Because Naltrexone works only on the beta-endorphin system, this experiment showed that sugar affects the brain the same way opioid drugs do, by stimulating a beta-endorphin release. Thanks to Dr. Blass, we now have solid scientific evidence that sugar works like a drug to block pain.

Sugar and Isolation Distress

In 1986, the year Blass did the experiments on sugar and physical pain, he also reported results from an experiment on sugar and emotional pain in which he measured the effect of sugar on "isolation distress." "Isolation distress" is a scientific term that describes the emotional stress of young animals when they are separated from their mothers and left alone.

Blass measured isolation distress in little mouse pups by measuring how many times they cried during the test period. When the pups were with Mama Mouse, they didn't cry. When they were taken away from Mama, they started crying big time. The eight pups that were given nothing to soothe them cried over 300 times in a six-minute period. The eight pups that were given sugar water cried only about 75 times in the same period. Next, Blass gave the pups a dose of Naltrexone before giving them sugar water, and as in the heat experiment the Naltrexone blocked the soothing effect of the sugar and the second batch of little pups cried as often as those who hadn't had the sugar. Apparently the sugar was blocking *emotional* pain just as it had blocked physical pain for the mice on the hot plate.

Since Blass's experiments, scientists have continued to look at the effects of sugar on the mind and body. Most of this work has been done in the context of alcoholism research. Since both sugar and alcohol evoke a beta-endorphin response, a number of studies have linked the preference for sweets to a preference for alcohol. Scientists have clearly shown that alcoholic mice—mice that have been bred to prefer alcohol—really go for sweets. The next step for science was to try these same experiments using people rather than mice.

In early 1997, Dr. Alexey Kampov-Polevoy published a study showing that alcoholic men much preferred a very sweet sugar drink (it was twice as sweet as Coke) to one which was less sweet. Only 16 percent of the nonalcoholics tested liked the very sweet drink best but more than two-thirds of the alcoholics did. We might well imagine that the alcoholics were having the same "Wow!" reaction to the sugar as Joe had to his first beer.

As scientists are slowly exploring the relationship of sugar to alcoholism, we can draw from our own experience as sugar-sensitive people to see how powerful a "drug" sugar can be. (Remember, a sugar-sensitive person has a significantly stronger beta-endorphin response to it than people with normal body chemistries.) We know how big an impact the soothing beta-endorphin release triggered by sugar has had on our own attitude toward sweet things. We seem to intuitively seek sugar when we need to quiet our physical and emotional pain. We also have the truth of our own pain-numbing experience with ice cream, chocolate, cereal and French bread. We didn't know it was caused by beta-endorphin, but we sure knew it was happening.

Why Not Sugar?

So, why not use sugar as a drug to ease our pain? "It's a food," you say. "What harm can there be in something so natural?" Stay with me, the story is still unfolding.

People with normal body chemistries experience the opioid effect of eating sugars as simply a pleasant feeling. For sugar-sensitive people, this pleasant feeling can become a euphoria which is powerful enough to create a strong attachment to the food or drink producing the effect. Because we love things that make us feel good, we want more. In fact, this heightened sensitivity to the druglike effects of sugar is the hallmark of the sugar-sensitive person.

Let's review why a sugar-sensitive person has such a powerful response to eating sugars. Remember that sugar-sensitive people have naturally low levels of beta-endorphin and their brains have opened up far more receptors to catch what little beta-endorphin there is. Because of this, sugar-sensitive people will have a heightened response to any substance that evokes beta-endorphin. Which is exactly what sugar and alcohol do.

This heightened response happens to Nancy when she eats ice cream. Nancy is sugar sensitive. Her natural levels of beta-endorphin are low. Most of the time she feels ugly, unacceptable, alone and generally out of touch with the world. But when she has ice cream, she feels really, really good: strong, safe and brave. So whenever Nancy feels upset, she just nestles down with a bowl of ice cream.

As she gets older, Nancy becomes dependent on the ice cream to maintain some semblance of feeling okay. But she is now quite overweight. So she commits to a diet and stops eating ice cream. For a little while she is pleased with her willpower. She starts to lose weight. But she doesn't feel good. She feels morbid, tearful and hopeless.

Then, before her period (beta-endorphin levels are at their lowest in women just before menstruation), Nancy starts feeling absolutely driven to get ice cream. She is sitting at her desk at work and the idea of chocolate chips and vanilla ice cream grabs her and won't let go. No, I am on a diet, she tells herself. Nancy goes home and her boyfriend calls. She is crabby. They have a fight. She gets into the car and drives to the convenience store at eleven at night. She buys a pint of Rocky Road ice cream and starts eating it in the car with a plastic spoon she keeps in her glove compartment. She feels much, much better. All is right with the world. For a little while. But as we will see, there will be a big price to pay for the comfort of the Rocky Road.

Cravings and Relapse

Aside from the havoc sweets cause in your blood sugar level, treats like ice cream, candy and other sugars can create a major problem for the sugar-sensitive person. The drug-induced "happiness" caused by these substances is short-lived and sets up cravings.

As we saw earlier, when you have low levels of serotonin, your brain produces cravings for simple carbohydrates, like sugar, that can be used to make more serotonin. In addition, cravings are closely linked to the beta-endorphin system.

Ingesting a small amount of a drug (like sugar) can make a person want more because of a mechanism in the beta-endorphin system called priming. Priming is the reason it is so hard for a sugar-sensitive person to "just say no" after having a taste of something sweet.

As we have seen, sweet foods or drinks activate a soothing beta-endorphin release. This is why candy has been recommended to alcoholics in early recovery. "It will cut your craving for alcohol," they are told. And that's true. Candy does cut alcohol cravings in the moment, but because it primes the beta-endorphin system to want more, it sets the person up for even stronger cravings—and alcohol relapse.

Minimizing the priming effect is a key part of stopping cravings. It is also a crucial part of relapse prevention. Priming an already upregulated beta-endorphin system will have a huge impact. Remember that after you stop using alcohol or sugar, your brain will open up even more beta-endorphin receptors to compensate for the reduction in beta-endorphin caused by going cold turkey. Because more receptors are open, an influx of beta-endorphin (triggered by the renewed use of sugar or alcohol) will have a huge impact.

If Nancy stops using sugar entirely and then one day decides to have dessert "just this once" at a business luncheon, she will feel wonderful. With so many receptors already waiting to receive the big influx of beta-endorphin, she will have an experience of euphoria that fairly sings to be repeated. If she isn't attentive to the priming effect of her "just this once" one dessert, she may find herself slipping back into her former big-time use of sugar.

Ice cream and chocolate do produce a wonderful sense of relaxation, but the sugar-sensitive person can become physically and emotionally dependent on them, and increasingly tolerant to their effects, be driven to eat more of them and experience withdrawal when they aren't used.

This pattern is addiction, plain and simple. Candy and ice cream are not pleasant and natural foods for the sugar-sensitive person. Even though they can help your brain produce serotonin, they are *not* the solution to either low serotonin levels or low beta-endorphin levels.

The Sugar-Sensitive Dilemma

So what are you to do? You are faced with two powerful dilemmas. You need carbohydrates to get tryptophan into your brain, and your naturally low level of beta-endorphin, which you inherited from your parents, gives you a heightened response to things that evoke a beta-endorphin response—things like ice cream, chocolate and alcohol.

Having these things makes you feel really good. They actually increase your feelings of self-esteem.

But when you eat sweet things (or drink alcohol) regularly, your beta-endorphin system downregulates over time, shutting down many of its receptors in an attempt to stem the influx of sugar-stimulated beta-endorphin and keep things on an even keel, so you need more sugar to get those good feelings. You end up feeling desperate. It has become even harder to stop because now you have withdrawal symptoms if you do.

Finally you decide to go cold turkey. You stop having alcohol or anything sweet and you weather feeling horrible for the first few weeks. You have managed to quiet the cravings and you feel better. But now your beta-endorphin system upregulates—it opens up more receptors so it can get more beta-endorphin, the influx of which has dropped since you cut out alcohol and sugar. This makes you a sitting duck for relapse. You have lots of receptors sitting there waiting to receive even a little alcohol or sugar and prime your brain with the message that beta-endorphin feelings are *good* and you should go get some more. If you decide to use sugar or alcohol when you are in this upregulated state, you will feel fantastic since you have lots of receptors to receive the beta-endorphin "feel-good" message. But when you try to stop again, it will be even more difficult than before because you now have more receptors open and waiting. More receptors mean greater withdrawal symptoms—more receptors screaming when their "drug" isn't there.

It becomes a vicious circle. After what you thought would be just a little bit of sugar or alcohol, your sugar-sensitive brain chemistry starts driving you to relieve the discomfort of these ever-greater withdrawal symptoms. Upregulation explains why we all have huge problems getting back on track after a slip in our diet or our sobriety.

If instead of quitting again, you keep on using a lot of chocolate, sugar or alcohol, your system will downregulate over time—close down some receptors—and you will have a harder and harder time receiving enough beta-endorphin. In as short a time as a few days, you will find yourself feeling worse. You keep hoping that you can find that wonderful feeling again, but it continues to elude you. You spend your life crawling through the days and trying to keep with-drawal at bay. You end up feeling like a true addict—you can't live with your drug and you can't live without it. And you think the whole thing is stupid because, after all, for goodness sakes, it's "just" sugar.

Balance Once Again

The story of sugar sensitivity has given you an explanation for the craziness you are feeling. But now you are ready for a solution. You want to feel better and medication like antidepressants isn't the an-swer. *It's not your fault.* This is a story about biochemistry. And there is an answer.

The solution is almost deceptively simple: *eat the right foods at the right times* and you can keep your serotonin and beta-endorphin at their optimal levels. The nutritional solution you'll learn is holistic, natural, fun, inexpensive and easy to follow. What's more, it has no side effects.

Eating the right food is the ideal way to keep your brain chemicals in balance all the time. Making food choices based on an understand-ing of how your brain and body chemistry work will prevent the dramatic ups and downs in beta-endorphin that lead to upregulation and downregulation, cravings and withdrawal symptoms.

In fact, by adjusting what you eat, you can deal with the three key issues of sugar sensitivity all at once: you can stabilize your blood sugar level, you can boost your beta-endorphin and serotonin levels, and you can minimize the dangerous priming effects. You don't have to cope with three different treatments, three different dosages or complex instructions. You don't even have to try to understand it all.

If you make some simple food changes, your body chemistry and brain chemistry will come into balance. You will reclaim your birth-right and feel energetic, optimistic, grounded, competent, easygoing and connected to others. You will also discover other ways to increase your body's natural production of beta-endorphin without using alcohol or sugar. Exercise, music, good sex, laughter, meditation, prayer, even the simple smell of an orange can all evoke beta-endorphin. We'll talk about each of these in later chapters. For now, all you need to remember is that there *is* life after addiction—and it's a very good life indeed.

Chapter 6

❂

Getting Started

Now that you have a good sense of the science behind sugar sensitivity, you are ready to put your food plan into action. As you do this, you will be the author of your own healing process. You will use the recommended tools to make changes in a way that will work for *you*. In my experience, the best preparation for change includes knowing your own style. Think about a time when you made a change in your life that really worked for you. How did you approach making that change?

One useful way to discover your style is to think about what you do when you're taking a trip to your favorite place. Do you just throw a toothbrush and some clean underwear in your bag and head out the door? Or do you go to AAA and get maps and guidebooks, make reservations for every stop along the way, trace your route with a pink marker, pack your bags three nights ahead and take along your first meal in a cooler? Or perhaps you call your travel agent, who handles it all and hands you an itinerary and your tickets.

Before you read any further, put your finger in the book right at this paragraph, then close your eyes and think about what you would do to get ready for a trip. Do you like to have a plan or do you explore things more spontaneously? Must you know all the facts or do you take things on trust? Do you prefer to do things all at once or do you take baby steps so that the process happens slowly?

Whatever you prefer, that's your personal style for making changes in your life. And a crucial part of your success with this program is adapting it to fit your own style. Although this program works much, much better if you take it slowly, it is important for you to start with what you've got—even if it's a preference to do things all at once. Each of you reading this book will go through the process slightly differently.

Don't Use the D-Word

Remember that developing a plan to address your sugar sensitivity isn't about going on a diet—it's about being in relationship with your food and your body. This means that you will have to learn to read your body, to hear what it is telling you. If you have been feeling "crazy" for a long time, it may seem hard to know what being healthy and balanced feels like. If so, turn to the charts in Chapter 3 and read over the words that describe what an optimal level of health feels like. Words like "energy," "focus," "stability" and "joy" will help you remember or imagine what is in store for you as you progress.

As you read the next chapters, you will learn what and when to eat to help you reach your goals. You will learn what you like, what triggers you, what makes you feel good, what makes you feel crazy, and what makes you feel clear. This is a *life plan* rather than a diet. You won't get a sheet that tells you in black and white exactly what to do. You will get guidelines and support on making the right choices for yourself. You will continually refine what works for you. Any slip you make will simply give you more information about your own vulnerabilities, about which biological system was activated or which brain chemical got out of balance.

Almost deceptively simple, the food plan you develop will address a number of complex systems all at once. As we move through the process, you also will learn how the positive changes you are making will affect each of the biochemical imbalances we have looked at. You will try out new behaviors and experience the resulting changes in your body. You will be able to see how these changes are in synch with the science of blood sugar and brain chemistry. Throughout the process, just let your body be your guide.

Now let's get started with your food plan.

Take It One Step at a Time

Your sugar-sensitive brain, with its love of impulsivity, may want you to do everything right away. "Give it to me all at once," it says. "Tell me the bottom line. Now!" You want to leap right in and give up alcohol, drugs, sugar and white flour—even caffeine and nicotine— right now. You want to get on with it.

Before you start, remember two critical points:

❏ **Don't try to do it all at once.**   ❏ **Take it in sequence.**

Yes, I know I told you to adapt the program to your own style, but these two things are critical to your success. Trust me.

First, don't try to do all seven steps all at once! Don't turn to Step 7 and start there. Do one step at a time. Do not proceed to the next step until you have mastered the one before it. Each step builds on the last. Don't skip around.

Some people ignore this advice and do what my client Tony did. He felt terrible when he first came to me. He had been trying to build up his body for six months by going to the gym to lose fat and add muscle. On a typical day Tony skipped breakfast and ate a power bar (a low-fat brand, of course) and an "energy charger" drink for lunch. Then he had a large plate of pasta for dinner with a huge salad. He drank a pot of coffee each day because it had no calories and gave him energy. In between his so-called meals, he snacked on candy for energy. He was exhausted most of the time. His muscles ached and he was on edge throughout the day.

When Tony and I talked, I outlined a plan that included spending a week doing Step 1 of my program—keeping a food journal—before he made any changes to his eating habits. But Tony wanted more. He left my office and decided he would stop eating sugar and drinking caffeine the next day. And he did. Three days later he had a severe migraine and felt as if he had been run over by a ten-ton truck, both of which are signs of sugar and caffeine withdrawal. It was clear to Tony that my program "didn't work."

The truth is that what Tony did doesn't work. If you try to do this program without following the steps sequence, it won't work. You will feel worse instead of better and you will give up.

If you do the steps in the recommended order, you will stabilize each of the biochemical functions involved in your sugar sensitivity. There is plenty of room in the plan for you to exercise your own judgment and make your own choices. But don't tinker with the big plan. Trust that there is a method to this madness. You will get dramatic results if you follow the plan as it's outlined. Done in that order, the program works.

The food plan that is presented is designed to change your blood chemistry and improve your neurotransmitter function. Even though it may seem obvious and simple, the foods in this plan create profound physical and emotional change. Don't be deceived by the simplicity. This is powerful medicine.

Seven Steps to Feeling Great

Here are the seven steps that will free you from the Dr. Jekyll/Mr. Hyde syndrome:

1. **Keeping a food journal**

2. **Eating three meals a day at regular intervals**

3. **Taking vitamins as recommended**

4. **Eating the recommended amount of protein at each meal**

5. **Adjusting your carbohydrate intake to include more complex foods**

6. **Reducing or eliminating sugars (including alcohol)**

7. **Creating a plan for maintenance**

Step 1: Keeping a Food Journal

The very first step in starting your program is keeping a record of the things you eat and drink—a food journal. Before you make any changes to your food, you need to understand your sugar-sensitive body and how it reacts to different foods. At this point, you may not know your own eating patterns. You may have nothing more than a general sense of how you feel. You might be able to remember having a good day or a bad day, but you can't say more than that.

The food journal helps you remember the details of each day. It provides a baseline for you at the beginning of your program. It gives you a picture of "before." As you continue the program, you will enjoy being able to look back at your journal and see how far you have come.

Your food journal will also teach you to read your own body. Your body doesn't have a computer printout to tell you directly what is going on with it, but it gives you clues and symptoms that hint at the bigger picture. These clues may not be in words, but your body talks in a consistent and predictable way. You just have to learn its language. Your food journal will teach you the language of your sugar-sensitive body.

Start by getting a blank book to write in. Find a book that you really like, one that fits your style and life rhythms. If you need to carry it with you, get one that fits in your pocket or purse. Go on a hunting expedition to find something perfect for you. Some people like to color in their journals or draw pictures. Molly used colored pens to highlight different foods in her journal. Jessica put her journal onto the computer and added to it each day. Mark drew lines under each entry. Elizabeth kept her journal right in her daily organizer. Let your journal fit who you are. Your journal will tell your story, so enjoy writing it. Don't skip this step. It is really, really important!

Once you have your own book to write in, keeping a food journal is very simple. First you make four columns. They will include:

1. The **date** and **time** of your entry.
2. **What you eat or drink.** Include amounts and be as specific as you can. Don't just write "chicken" and "potato." Put down

"one large roasted chicken breast" and "one huge baked potato with 2 tablespoons of sour cream." If you don't know weights or measurements, it will help to learn them. Get a set of measuring cups and spoons. You might even buy a food scale. You don't need to be precise, but your estimates should be in the ballpark. Experiment so that you can begin to estimate reasonably well.

Learn the difference between 1 and 2 cups of milk or between 4 and 10 ounces of meat. Reading labels will also give you a sense of the amounts you are eating. Remember to write down what you drink as well. Include things like milk, soda, juice or alcohol. Also include the amount of water you drink. Water helps to keep your system clean.

3. **How you feel physically.** Write down anything you notice about how you feel. Physical symptoms are body sensations. There is a huge range of physical symptoms. They can reflect a state of imbalance or a state of balance. You may not have noticed these symptoms specifically before. The more you pay attention, the more useful your food journal will become. The chart which follows will show you some feelings:

Clues for Imbalance	Clues for Balance
Headaches	Bright eyes
Stomach pain	Hunger
Muscle cramps	Stamina
Coughing	Natural deep breathing
Fatigue	High energy
Insomnia	Restful sleep
Restlessness	Focus
Shakiness	Alertness
Muscle weakness	Strength
No concentration	Good attention span
Pallor	Good color

4. **How you feel emotionally.** Pay attention to what you are feeling. You may have a hard time with this one. Some people write "fine" or "good" for many pages. Use the list below to help you learn to describe different kinds of feelings:

Clues for Imbalance	Clues for Balance
Anxious	Confident
Bored	Excited
Scared	Energized
Mad	Humorous
Sad	Happy
Depressed	Interested
Scattered	Focused
Restless	Calm
Irritable	Relaxed
Agitated	Easygoing
Hyper	Patient

Here is an example of what a blank page of a food journal might look like:

Date Time	What I Ate or Drank	How I Feel Physically	How I Feel Emotionally

How the Food Journal Works

Go ahead and start your own journal. Write down what you eat or drink. Try to write it down as soon as you have eaten something rather than waiting until the end of the day. Write down physical or emotional feelings whenever you notice them, not just when you eat. For example, you may find that you feel really good at lunchtime, then at 1:30 P.M. you feel as if you would like to lie down and go to sleep. Write down what you had for lunch at 12:30 P.M. and then write down "Sleepy" at 1:30 P.M. Carry your book with you. The more specific and detailed your journal, the more information you will have to work with in creating your own food plan.

You may find that getting started with your journal is easy but continuing is difficult. Sometimes people want to do the program but remain resistant to the idea of keeping a food journal. Often, they have no idea why. You may think it's too much trouble or you can't be bothered. You may start with a bang and then fizzle out in a few days: "I didn't remember to take my book with me," "Writing it all down got too bothersome," "I lost it," "I know what I eat, I don't have to write it down."

Sometimes people really do not want to look at how they eat. Writing things down seems terrifying or petty. You may have feelings of failure or hopelessness attached to the way you eat. Even the idea of a food journal may make you panic. You may be surprised to discover that food has a bigger emotional charge for you than you realized. You may have had bad experiences with writing down your food.

Some diet programs require you to keep a log in which you record everything you eat. You are allowed only a certain number of units of bread or meat or fruit, so recording your food becomes a way of seeing whether you have been "bad" and eaten more than you were supposed to. This approach can set up a real feeling of deprivation and thus make the food log the target of your frustration or resentment. The log reinforces the negative feelings you may already have about yourself and your relationship to food.

The program I have developed helps you change these old beliefs

—and any others that get in the way of making changes in your life. The process is designed to be fun, informative and free of negative judgments. If negative feelings come up, if you feel bad about writing down that you ate three jelly doughnuts at 9 A.M., remember that you are recording information that will help you later see the connection between what you eat and how you'll feel emotionally and physically.

If you find that you keep your food journal for a few days and then forget to do it, write that down in your journal. Keep track of what-

Date & Time	What I Ate or Drank	How I Feel Physically	How I Feel Emotionally
Nov. 10			
7:00	2 doughnuts	Tired	Depressed. Feel as if I can hardly function
11:00	2 cups of coffee with cream and sugar		Really good
11:15		Exhausted	Crabby about work
1:00	Burrito		
1:15	Nachos	Unable to stay awake	
	Large Coke	Wired	Sad. How can I be wired and sad at the same time?
3:15	2 cups of coffee with cream and sugar	Relaxed	Happy
4:00		Tense	Satisfied
5:30	3 beers	Relaxed	
7:00	3 pieces of chicken, coleslaw, mashed potatoes, 2 biscuits with butter and honey, hot fudge sundae with whipped cream and nuts	Warm	Feel great!
8:00		Full	

ever comes up for you for *at least a week*. Even if you end up with six pages that say you forgot to notice, keep writing!

The table opposite is a sample page from a beginning food journal. Take a look at it to get a sense of what you can put in yours.

Using Your Journal as a Planning Tool

At the end of a week, take a look at what you've written in your food journal. Do not criticize what you ate. Simply look at the facts. You are doing Step 1 now and it doesn't matter if you eat only chocolate for three weeks, or if you have been eating ice cream every night at 11 P.M., or if you have been skipping two out of three meals.

Go back to the very first page and look over your entries for the last week. Without judgment, pay attention to what you see. Go back over what you have written and try to remember each day and each meal. Don't try to figure out what it means. Don't jump ahead and try to analyze everything.

Now examine the times when you ate. Take a separate piece of paper and write down a summary showing the dates and the times you ate. Don't include what foods you ate or how you felt. Your paper will look something like this:

10/12	11:00 A.M.	breakfast
	3:00 P.M.	snack
	6:30 P.M.	dinner
	10:30 P.M.	snack
10/13	12:30 P.M.	lunch
	2:30 P.M.	snack
	8:30 P.M.	dinner
	10:00 P.M.	snack
	11:00 P.M.	snack
10/14	1:30 P.M.	lunch
	3:00 P.M.	beer
	6:00 P.M.	drinks
	9:00 P.M.	snack

Becoming a Good Detective

After you have made this summary, write out the answers to the questions which follow. Answer every question carefully. Proceed like a detective on the hunt for information about your sugar-sensitive body.

Do you eat at mealtimes?
Do you eat between meals?
Do you graze throughout the day?
Do you eat at the same times each day?
How long do you wait to eat?

Write about what you have discovered. Take some time to reflect on your pattern. Let the answer to each of the questions sink in. You will begin to see your patterns of eating. Don't judge yourself. The more you are able to just observe and note these things, the easier it will be for you to make changes later.

Looking at Your Eating Patterns

Let's take a look at each of these questions more closely:

❑ **Do you eat at mealtimes?** Which times of the day do you eat? Do you eat at regular mealtimes or do you eat whenever you remember to get around to it? Typical mealtimes are seven in the morning, noon and six in the evening. Mealtimes may vary in different families, but generally include one meal in the morning reasonably soon after getting up, one meal at midday and one meal in the evening. It is often a surprise for sugar-sensitive people to see how irregularly they eat. Or they may have a regular routine during the week and then change everything on the weekend.

❑ **Do you eat between meals?** Even if you eat regular meals, you may eat between mealtimes, too. You may get hungry before your next meal or you may eat because you feel tired, bored, restless or upset. You may eat because everyone at work does. You may eat just because food is there. Nurses often talk about having candy all day long because the patients at the hospital always keep the nursing station in good supply.

❑ **Do you graze throughout the day?** Some people don't eat meals. They catch what they can as they're working. You might find you are really busy at work and can't take the time to eat a meal. You eat a little as you go. Or you may have children at home and really don't have time to sit down for a meal. Sometimes people just need to have food with them. They carry a little snack as they go throughout the day.

❑ **Do you eat at the same times each day?** How regularly do you eat? You may eat three times a day but always at different times. Your work shift may change or you may find that you simply don't notice the clock. You eat only when you notice you are hungry. Or you eat when you get around to it. At what intervals do you eat? Some people wait until they fall off the cliff from low blood sugar and then eat. How long it takes to fall off the cliff depends on what they had to eat at their last meal.

❑ **How long do you wait to eat?** Notice how long you are able to go before you simply have to eat something. Some people never get hungry. They actually feel better if they don't eat. Others can't go more than a few hours. Others have very consistent and regular eating intervals but they never even think about it.

After you have done this exercise, you should be able to describe your eating pattern in a clear summary.

Looking at What You Eat

After you have become really familiar with your style of eating, look at the content of your eating. Set aside your date-and-time summary and go back to your complete food journal. Look at what foods you are actually eating at meals and for snacks, then answer these questions:

What kinds of foods do you usually eat?
How much sweet food do you eat?

Are you eating any protein?

Are you drawn to fat?

Are you using a lot of caffeine?

Go through these questions in the same way that you did those for when you eat.

❏ **What kinds of foods do you usually eat?** What foods are you drawn to? Many people who are sugar sensitive eat mostly carbohydrates such as bread, sweets and pasta. Or they like lots of fruit. Can you get a sense of your main staple? Do you see anything appearing every day? Look for patterns.

❏ **How much sweet food do you eat?** Try taking a yellow marker and highlighting the sweet foods you recorded in your journal. This will provide you with visual confirmation of whether you are drawn to sweet foods. Sugar-sensitive people often eat sweets two or three times a day. Do you nibble as you go? Or do you binge on sweets? Do you have them every day? Get to know your own sweet-tooth pattern. Remember that sweets come in two forms. The first is overt sugars like candy, soda, cookies or cake. The second is covert sugars such as the high-fructose cornstarch found in many processed foods or the hidden sugar in canned vegetables or ketchup. You have to read labels with a fine-tooth comb to find the coverts. (We'll talk a lot more about this in Chapter 9.)

❏ **Are you eating any protein?** Protein is found in eggs, milk, cheese, yogurt, meat, fish, chicken, beans, seeds, nuts and many grains. Look to see if and when you are eating proteins. Are they a regular part of your diet? Are you drawn to them? Do you consciously choose them or do you try to avoid them?

❏ **Are you drawn to fat?** Fat, like sugar, is linked to the beta-endorphin system. Sugar-sensitive people may well have an increased opioid response to eating fat. Fat and sugar work in tandem. If you've cut down on your fat, you may have unwittingly added a lot of sugars. Likewise, if you eat less sugar, pay attention in your food journal to how and when you add fat. Moderate levels of fat can work in your behalf because they will not spike your blood sugar.

❑ **Are you using a lot of caffeine?** Notice how often you have something which contains caffeine. This may include coffee, tea, chocolate and certain sodas like Coke, Pepsi, Mountain Dew, Dr Pepper and Jolt. Some over-the-counter medications like NoDoz, Vivarin and Vanquish contain caffeine. Do you find that you use caffeine at a regular time each day? Notice how you feel before and after you have the caffeine.

Assessing Where You Stand

Now that you are becoming familiar with your food journal, fill out this questionnaire. Check the box that applies to you. Score one if

	Yes	No
1. I use alcohol.	0	1
2. I eat three meals a day at regular intervals.	1	0
3. I eat protein at each meal.	1	0
4. I eat approximately the recommended amount of protein each day (.4 gram × my weight in pounds).	1	0
5. I use caffeine in: ☐ coffee ☐ tea ☐ soda. Indicate how much you drink a day.	0	1
6. I eat overt sugars (table sugar, cake, cookies, ice cream, candy, etc.).	0	1
7. I eat covert sugars (sugars such as high-fructose corn syrup hidden in food).	0	1
8. I eat foods made with refined white flour, such as bread and pasta.	0	1
9. I smoke cigarettes (__per day).	0	1
10. I take a B-complex vitamin, vitamin C and at least 15 mg of zinc daily.	1	0
	Total	

the box you checked has a 1 in it and score zero if the box has a 0 in it. You will probably need two to three weeks of data to see all of your typical patterns. We have not talked about all of these issues yet, but they will give you a sense of the total program.

Add up your score. Get your food journal and double-check your answers. Let's go through them together.

1. I use alcohol. If you ever have something alcoholic to drink, even if you drink only once a month, the answer will be yes. Check no if you have made an intentional decision not to drink alcohol or to remain clean and sober, and you have stuck to your decision, or if you simply don't drink. As we saw in Chapters 3 and 4, drinking alcohol increases your blood sugar level and negatively affects your beta-endorphin system.

2. I eat three meals a day at regular intervals. A meal includes two or more nutritious foods at a sitting. A bagel and coffee does not count as a meal. A hot fudge sundae does not count as a meal. A bagel and a scrambled egg would be a meal. A tuna fish sandwich and an apple could be a meal. Do you eat three meals a day every day during an entire week? If you skipped any days during the week, answer this question no. Regular intervals means that you eat your meals between four and six hours apart. Traditional mealtimes of 7 A.M., noon and 6 P.M. provide a reasonable guide for regular intervals.

3. and 4. I eat the recommended amount of protein at each meal. Protein foods are eggs, milk, cheese, yogurt, meat, fish, chicken, beans, seeds, nuts and many grains. If you do not eat enough protein at each meal, or if you do not eat three meals a day, or if you eat more than the recommended amount (.4 gram × your body weight in pounds), then the answer to these questions will also be no.

5. I use caffeine. Caffeine is found in coffee, tea, hot cocoa, Coke, Diet Coke, Royal Crown Cola, Mountain Dew, Dr Pepper, chocolate, chocolate candy, NoDoz, Midol, Bromo-Seltzer, etc. (a full list is found in Chapter 11). Because caffeine is an addictive substance that can affect your mood and may create problems, we will want to take a look later at your caffeine use.

6. I eat overt sugars. Overt sugars are cake, candy, ice cream, soda and things that you traditionally think of as sweets.

7. I eat covert sugars. Covert sugars are the sweet things hidden in foods, like high-fructose corn syrup, malt barley, maltodextrin, concentrated pear juice, white grape juice and raisin paste. Fruit is a covert sugar. Most people are not aware of covert sugars until they start reading labels. If you have not made a conscious choice to eliminate sugars from your diet, you are probably eating covert sugars. We will talk about covert sugars in depth in Chapter 9.

8. I eat foods made with refined white flour. These foods include white bread, refined-flour breads, white rice, French bread, bagels, pastry and pasta.

9. I smoke cigarettes. If you smoke at all (even two cigarettes a month), answer this question yes.

10. I take a B-complex vitamin, vitamin C and at least 15 mg of zinc daily. The recommended vitamin protocol explained in Chapter 7 includes these. If you are not taking them, the answer will be no. If you are taking megavitamins or supplements that don't contain the amounts recommended, the answer will be no.

Your Score

As you start your new food plan, your total score will probably be between zero and 3. Don't be discouraged. The lower your score is, the more dramatic your results will be. Your score will change over time. As people change their eating habits with this plan, their scores move up to 5 or 6. When their scores progress to 7 or 8, they feel wonderful. The increase in your score will give you a good reading on how you are progressing.

If your score is higher than 3, you have already started to make changes which will support your recovery. Even if you score an 8 or 9, you will find the information which follows a useful support to your program.

By now, you should be well on your way to keeping a complete food journal. Congratulations! And keep your food journal going as you move through the next six steps of your program.

Chapter 7

✪

Take Three Giant Steps

Now that you understand the vital role of your food journal, you can start to work with food itself. Working with the food (please note I do not mean dieting) may evoke feelings of deprivation: "Oh, no, you aren't going to take away my ice cream, are you?" Or sugar or coffee or French bread or whatever you are most attached to. Starting to work with food is likely to touch some pretty core feelings.

Please remember that my program is based on an *abundance* model rather than a *deprivation* model. I am not taking away anything. At some point you may decide that you do not want to eat foods that contribute to your "craziness." But *you* will be making that decision from a place where you feel filled up, nourished and committed to your health.

To get to that place, we start not by taking foods away, but by adding them.

We will look again at the seven steps. The steps we will be covering in this chapter are highlighted.

Let's move to Steps 2, 3 and 4. Remember you will be continuing your food journal throughout your program. As you do Steps 2, 3 and 4, you'll be pleased to notice that you start to feel better quickly, even before you've begun to reduce the sugars you eat. Don't jump ahead, don't skip and don't leave any of these early steps out. The plan works as a sequence.

Step 2: Eating Three Meals a Day at Regular Intervals

The second step for you to take is to eat three meals every day at regular intervals. This means eating nutritious food every day. The good news is that to master Step 2 you don't have to make any other changes in your food. You don't have to stop eating pasta or chocolate. You don't have to eliminate espresso. Just move whatever you *are* eating to a mealtime. If you have been going out for ice cream in the evening, you can keep eating the ice cream—just make sure you eat it with a meal. If you have been eating M&M's every day, you can continue to eat them if you like—just eat them with a meal.

A "meal" is eating two or more nutritious foods at one sitting. Tuna fish and salad or eggs and toast would be a meal. My clients have asked if a hot fudge sundae is a meal. "What if we add a banana and more nuts?" they say. That is stretching it. But at this stage of the game, trust yourself to identify two or more nutritious foods.

I do not encourage snacking for sugar-sensitive people because all too often snacking can lead to "grazing." Grazing happens when you eat your way through the day. People are often encouraged to eat this way in order to maintain a steady level of sugar in the blood. However, for someone with a sugar-sensitive or addictive body chemistry, snacking can create trouble. Grazing reinforces a lack of impulse control, which is already a problem for people with naturally low serotonin: if they get hungry, they eat right away rather than wait. Learning to start and then *stop* a meal is a very good behavior change for the sugar-sensitive person.

Eating at regular intervals will ensure that your blood sugar doesn't drop to a crisis point. If you do not go longer than five or six hours before you have your next meal, you are not likely to get into the danger zone. Paying attention to having your meals at regular intervals also helps you pay attention to your food and your body—one of our goals in your program.

The Magic of Breakfast

Many of the people I have worked with have balked at eating breakfast. "I don't feel hungry in the morning," they say. "Should I eat if I don't feel hungry?" The answer is yes. A normal, chemically balanced body uses hunger as a cue to inform its owner that it needs more fuel. People who are sugar sensitive usually do not live in a state of chemical balance. Because of this, you don't get the physiological cues that other people do. All bodies need food after a period of fasting, such as the time from dinner to breakfast. If you don't feel hungry in the morning, it's because your thermostat is not working properly.

Once you start to eat breakfast regularly, you may also begin feeling hungry in the morning. This is a good sign. It means your body is starting to regain its chemical balance. You may also find that you feel a whole lot better right away. Many people are amazed at what a difference eating breakfast makes in how they feel.

Sometimes people get scared because they experience all sorts of feelings when they get hungry in the morning. They are afraid that if they are hungry first thing, they will eat, and if they eat, they will gain weight and get (or stay) fat. Not eating allows them to feel safe, in control. When they add breakfast and start to feel hungry in the morning, it threatens their old feeling of safety and they want to quit the whole program.

The important thing is to take it slowly. You don't have to spook yourself. You are simply trying to master the food journal and eat

three meals a day. If breakfast is hard for you, look around and see if
there is anything you might use to start with. Remember that "breakfast" can be as creative as you are.

You can eat the foods traditionally associated with breakfast, such
as cereal and juice, or you can experiment with foods you may never
have thought of for breakfast, like burritos, a bowl of soup or a baked
potato. If you do not have a problem with cholesterol, try having
one or two eggs in the morning. Eggs have very high nutrition, and
sugar-sensitive people usually respond very well to them.

If you still have a problem with the idea of food first thing in the
morning, you can try making a power shake that consists of milk,
juice, oatmeal and some protein powder (recipe on page 114). Often
this is an easy and manageable beginning for the breakfast hater. If
you try this, use fresh fruit or frozen juice that is unsweetened, and
choose a protein powder that has no sugars and provides more than
20 grams of protein in 2 tablespoons.

When you buy protein powder—and other foods for this plan—
be aware that sugar is often disguised by other names. (See Chapter 8
for a complete list of sugar's many aliases.) Also remember that a food
manufacturer may call something sugar-free as long as it does not
contain sucrose, which is only one of the many kinds of sugars.

You can use milk in your shake if you like the taste. Choose the
type of milk which best suits you. Using lactose-free milk will reduce
the sugars content. If you prefer not to use milk in your power shake,
you can substitute diluted fruit juice at the rate of 6 ounces of water
to 3 ounces of juice. Many people I know use the complex carbohydrate drink Mill Milk, an oat-based product that has no added sugar
and tastes wonderful. You can also use soy milk products, but be sure
to read the labels first because soy milk may have a great deal of
sweetener added in the form of barley or rice syrup.

Don't be afraid to experiment. If your mother told you that you
can't possibly have chili or pizza for breakfast, remember that your
mother isn't in charge of your meals anymore. If you want chili or
pizza for breakfast, eat it and enjoy! You're on your way to creating
your own food plan, one that fits your needs today as a unique,
sugar-sensitive person.

Here are some of the foods my clients eat for breakfast. Make up your own list of choices that work for you. Share ideas with your friends. Finding new ideas for breakfast can become an interesting treasure hunt.

Great Ideas for Breakfast

- 2 eggs, 1 slice of whole grain toast and ½ cup orange juice
- 1½ cups cooked oatmeal mixed with 2 tablespoons protein powder, plus a little milk or cream, decaf coffee
- Veggie burger and salad
- ¾ cup cottage cheese and ½ cup strawberries
- 2 slices of whole grain toast with peanut butter
- Corned beef hash with 1 egg and whole grain toast
- Power shake
- Breakfast burrito with whole wheat tortilla, eggs, beans, cheese
- 2 eggs and 1 orange
- 1 cup of chili and brown rice
- Scrambled tofu and vegetables
- Whole grain waffle with protein powder in the batter, applesauce and yogurt on top

---

"How Much Should I Eat?"

You may be wondering how much food you are supposed to eat at your three meals a day. "Where are the tables?" you may ask. "Where are the exchange lists?"

There aren't any. You will sort this out as part of the process. If you are a small person, eat less. If you are a big person, eat more. At the end of your meal, you should feel comfortably full but not stuffed.

Many people get nervous when they aren't told exactly what to do. But if I tell you everything to do, then you are just listening to my instructions rather than trusting your own ability to find what is right for you. Experiment. Try different amounts. You'll find that too little won't work and too much will make you gain weight. *Listen to your body.* Use all that experience you've packed away over the years.

If you have a problem with compulsive eating, have an eating disorder like anorexia or bulimia, or are eating large amounts of sugar and caffeine, your body probably won't know what the right amount is. Simply work with learning to eat three meals a day. Sometimes this step takes months to master. That's okay.

What's a "Regular Interval"?

Your meals need to be no more than five or six hours apart. Typical mealtimes are 7 A.M., noon and 6 P.M. But your schedule may require something quite different. If you work a night shift or your work keeps you tied up through standard mealtimes, you may have to adjust your eating times.

But don't eat breakfast at 6 A.M., wait until 2 P.M. for lunch and then eat dinner at 10 P.M. If this is your normal pattern, however, and you know you won't change it, then find a way to live with it. You will have to get yourself a healthy snack in between lunch and dinner. Drink a power shake midmorning if you need to. Carry a snack that includes protein: apples and cheese, nuts and fruit, or peanut butter and a banana. Whatever appeals to you. But feed your body more often. You shouldn't go more than six hours without food except between dinner and breakfast the next morning. Your blood sugar will drop too low and you will become tired, frustrated and irritable. Your concentration will suffer—and so will your work.

It may sound as if there is a contradiction here. First I say, "Avoid snacking," then I recommend it. Let me clarify. The best option for sugar-sensitive people is to eat three meals a day at regular intervals without snacks in between. When you eat regular meals and don't "graze" you teach your addictive body the new behavior of starting and *stopping*. However, I am a practical woman. I know that some people won't be able to eat that way. That's why I present the other option: snacks with protein. It is better for you to know you have another option if you have to use it. This food plan is designed to support you in finding what *works* for you, not in making you work for it.

So that's Step 2: eat three meals a day and eat them no more than five or six hours apart. It sounds simple, but it can be a challenge if this has not been your pattern. And remember that until you get the stability that comes from eating three meals a day at regular intervals, your food plan won't work long term. Don't be fooled into thinking that this part is so easy you don't have to work on it. If you are sugar sensitive, Step 2 is the key to getting your body chemistry in balance.

Step 3: Taking Vitamins as Recommended

Many addiction-recovery programs recommend megavitamins or huge amounts of amino acids. Clients often come to me expecting to go home with a long list of supplements to take. They are surprised when I talk about food rather than supplements.

People with addictive bodies love to take something, be it pills, white powder or special mixtures from a can. Taking something becomes the solution rather than creating a lifestyle with a healthy relationship to food. I am careful not to reinforce this mode of thinking. Eating food as your solution to sugar sensitivity demands that you think about what food you will eat, when, how and with whom. Eating food moves you into the relational aspects of your recovery.

With that said, I also recommend a simple vitamin protocol because it will speed your body in its return to balance. Vitamin C, a B-complex vitamin and zinc are traditionally used in alcohol detox. Since sugar sensitivity is so closely linked to the metabolic pathways of alcoholism, I encourage the use of the same vitamins in this food plan. In the course of this plan, you will be doing a detox yourself. Over time you will be moving away from the more refined foods, reducing your sugar and alcohol intake, and avoiding junk food.

Vitamin C speeds detoxification and acts as a scavenger that consumes free radicals, which are the destructive by-products of toxin activity within your body. Vitamin C helps your adrenals recover from adrenal fatigue. Finally, vitamin C helps your brain chemicals work properly by supporting the conversion of the amino acid tryptophan (found in the protein you eat) into serotonin.

The B vitamins are essential in breaking down carbohydrates so the body can burn them as fuel. One of the B vitamins, niacin, is critical to the conversion of tryptophan into serotonin. Many of the other B vitamins do other useful things which will not be discussed here. I do not want you to start experimenting with taking lots of separate B vitamins to "maximize" the particular effect you are seeking. This is what addicts do—play around with the variables to get the best punch possible. I want to reinforce the holistic approach. So I recommend you take a B-vitamin complex.

Zinc is a mineral that has a number of beneficial effects in recovery. They are all quite complicated and work at a very subtle level to enable insulin to do its job and help digest the food you eat, among other functions. It isn't necessary for you to know the details. Just trust me when I say that zinc will help your recovery process.

You will need to learn a bit about these vitamins to determine a dosage that fits your needs. I can—and will—tell you what ranges of dosage I have used with my clients, but because there are so many conflicting claims about vitamins I recommend that you talk to your health practitioner or a person skilled in nutrition about your specific lifestyle and current eating patterns.

An appropriate vitamin C dosage may vary from 500 to 5000 mg a day. The doctors skilled in vitamin C supplementation often suggest a "bowel tolerance" dosage. That means starting low and adding a little more vitamin C each day. If you find yourself having gas, diarrhea or stomach distress, cut your dosage back by 500 mg at a time until the symptoms subside. Vitamins C and B are both water soluble, so drinking plenty of water will help minimize any overload of these vitamins. What isn't used will simply be washed out of your body.

Always take the B vitamins in a complex form so that you get the right proportions of them. Taking the B vitamins in a liquid form will allow you to experiment with different amounts to find what is the best dosage for you. Here is one place your addictive side can have the fun of experimenting with the dosage—within a specifically defined time period. B-complex formulas usually come in dosages of 25, 50, 75 or 100. Read the label. A teaspoon of the liquid is a 50. Do not take more than a 50 in a given day. And do not take B vitamins at night as they may keep you awake. If you feel at all jittery, take less.

The recommended dosage of zinc is 15 to 25 mg a day. If you suck zinc lozenges to prevent a cold, pay attention to the dosage in each lozenge. Do not take more than 30 mg in a given day.

As I said earlier, don't take megadose supplements (i.e., vitamins and minerals) or amino acid supplements. This approach reinforces the idea of "taking something" to "fix it," which is precisely the kind of behavior you want to replace. You may have used drugs, alcohol, sugar or French bread to help you "fix" your "crazy" feelings.

Whether a person is in drug, alcohol or sugar detox, the brain is in a vulnerable state during the transition to being drug-free. This compromised state might politely be called mush brain. In my experience, people in detox can effectively keep no more than three things in mind at the same time. This is why three meals and three vitamins make a good package. The times of active substance use or substance withdrawal are not the best times to follow a food plan that is complex and requires a huge amount of calculation. You may get to complexity later, but at the beginning strive for simplicity, simplicity, simplicity.

The Bigger Picture

The vitamins you start taking in Step 3 will be helpful, but don't forget that the most crucial element of this program is eating *food*. Food provides vitamins naturally and promotes healing. Preparing food and meals provides much more than that. Buying, preparing and eating nutritious food requires specific behavior changes and makes you become conscious about what you are eating. Most people who have relied on sugar for a long time have very little experience with the type of behavioral change required for planning meals. Doing your food plan calls for you to make plans for regular meals and follow through on them. It means learning to devise alternative plans of action (like figuring out what and when to eat when your schedule suddenly changes), which reinforces flexibility and creative problem-solving. Doing a full food plan rather than just taking vitamins and hoping they will make you healthy also teaches you to make discriminating judgments about what is good specifically for you. All of these things are incredibly self-empowering.

As you will see, what you initiate with the food plan will have a far bigger impact than just eating three times a day. You will learn to pay attention to your body in a consistent way and make a connection between how you feel and what you are eating. As your food gets stable, you will become more and more interested in what works for your body and your needs. As you eat three meals a day at regular intervals and take your vitamins, you may find yourself getting impatient. This happened with a client of mine named Mary.

Mary had been doing her food journal and eating three meals pretty much every day. But she was getting impatient. She wanted to go faster—to do the rest of the steps right away. She was even ready to completely stop using sugar, she told me. And couldn't she also stop using caffeine now? she asked. Mary felt she had done Steps 1 and 2. She didn't want to keep her food journal anymore because she was eating three meals most days. She wanted to be in charge of her own plan.

Mary presented me with a dilemma. I wanted to support her in taking charge of her own process but at the same time I knew from my work with other clients how important it is to follow the steps in sequence. I stuck to my guns. I encouraged Mary to continue her food journal and master having three meals every single day before she made any other changes. I knew that doing this would create the stability Mary needed for making the changes called for in Steps 3 through 7. Skip the first two steps—or stop doing them—and the process will not work.

Remember, it absolutely does not matter how long it takes to master each of these steps.

You, like Mary, will get to negotiate the order in which you make change after you have done the first three steps. But *always* begin with the journal and keep doing it. It is your key to understanding where you started. Without a food journal, the process is just talk. It is a waste of your time to try to do the whole program and the changes it involves without doing the journal. You will not have to do a journal forever, but having it by your side as you master your food plan adds a crucial and powerful tool to your work.

Step 4: Eating Protein with Each Meal

The next step is for you to eat protein at every meal. Protein provides the raw materials to help your brain and body heal. Most important for you, protein provides the tryptophan your body needs to make serotonin, which keeps you feeling calm, productive, creative and competent.

Protein also helps to slow down your digestion. Proteins are very, very complex foods and your body has to work hard to break them down into a simple form that can best be used. They also help to stabilize your blood sugar levels so you won't have the steep peaks and valleys that can be so disastrous for sugar-sensitive people.

Before we go into which foods contain protein, let's take a look at how protein works. Protein is made up of amino acids, which are the building blocks for thousands of cell functions. Your body needs twenty different amino acids to function properly. They are used to make digestive enzymes, to maintain the fluid balance in your body, to make the antibodies which protect you against disease, to make hormones such as thyroid and insulin, to build things like bones and teeth, and to help your eyes respond to light. Needless to say, protein is important.

Some of these amino acids can be produced in the body. Others, called essential amino acids, must be provided by the food you eat. A food, like beef, that contains all the essential amino acids is called a complete protein.

Giving your body complete proteins is important. Eating any type of protein will raise the amount of amino acids in your bloodstream. But in order for these amino acids to get into your cells and do their job, you must either eat complete proteins that contain all of the essential amino acids or you must make sure that your diet includes the plant protein foods which complement one another.

Proteins derived from animal foods (meat, fish, eggs and dairy products) are complete, while proteins derived from plants (vegetables, beans and grains) are generally not complete. If you are a vegetarian and choose to eat only plant proteins, it is important to combine them to make sure your body gets all of the essential amino acids. For example, rice and beans or soy and oats each contain incomplete proteins. But if you eat both, they provide all of the essential amino acids your body needs. You do not need to eat the complementary proteins at the same time. The balance over the entire day is more important. You can find information about food combinations in a number of vegetarian and other cookbooks. A number of myths have continued about the inadequacy of plant proteins or about the need for strict complementation at each meal. Current thinking suggests that if you are eating enough regular food and obtaining an adequate amount of total protein, it is very likely that all the needs for amino acid complementation will be met.

Foods with Protein

Here are some foods containing protein:

Eggs	Poultry
	Chicken, turkey, game hens, ostrich, pheasant, duck, goose
Fish	**Meats**
White fish, crab, lobster, clams, tuna, swordfish, cod, salmon, mackerel, trout and many others	Beef, pork, veal, lamb, venison, buffalo, rabbit, goat
Dairy	**Beans/Grains/Nuts/Seeds**
Milk, cheese, yogurt, cottage cheese	Tofu, tempeh, lentils, kidney beans, all other beans; quinoa, amaranth, millet, other grains; peanut butter, almond butter, any other nut butters

The USDA recommended daily allowance (RDA) of protein for a 150-pound adult is 54 grams a day, or a little less than 0.4 gram per pound of body weight. I recommend that sugar-sensitive people on my program eat a little more than that. A good guideline is to have between .4 and .6 gram per pound of body weight depending on your health needs. In the early stages of your recovery, your body may have more repair work to do and you may need to eat more protein. Later, as you feel better, you can reduce the amount.

Many people ask me for the exact number of grams of protein they should eat. Counting grams is a tradition that has come from counting calories or grams of fat. I actually discourage focusing on an exact count because counting grams puts the focus on the measurement rather than the relationship to what you are eating.

Although diet and nutrition books show the amount of protein in a specific serving of food in grams, it may be easier for you to convert this to ounces when you are planning your meals. Seven grams of protein equals an ounce of animal protein foods. If you weigh 150 pounds, you will be having a minimum of 8 to 9 ounces (56 to 63 grams) of animal protein (such as beef, chicken and lamb) each day.

Remember, though, this does not mean that having an 8-ounce steak for dinner fulfills your protein requirement. The daily protein should be broken up into three servings, one at each meal. Eating a huge amount of protein at one time creates a lot of work for your body since it takes a lot of work to break down. Don't make your body suffer by trying to do it all at once. "All or nothing" is also what people with addictive bodies do.

If you have lots of experience measuring grams and portions, calculating your protein intake may be familiar to you. However, trying to measure grams, kilograms or even ounces can be intimidating for some people. Particularly in the early stages of your recovery, you may find it hard to pay attention to this level of detail.

If this is true, there is an easier alternative. Hold out your hand and make a fist. Look at your fist and use that size portion to figure out how much protein you will be eating at each meal. A big fist means you need more protein than if you had a little fist. You will always have your measuring tool with you. The average-size fist translates into two eggs, one medium chicken breast, one medium-size hamburger patty, a round ball of tuna fish or a cereal bowl–size serving of lentils. Get the idea? Good. And remember, it is more important to eat protein regularly than to have a rigid measurement or portion at each meal.

You may find it helpful to make a food serving/protein chart for yourself which lists the foods you are most likely to eat. Here is the

chart Margot made for herself to show some sample protein choices
for a meal:

2 eggs	1 small container yogurt
2 tablespoons protein powder	4 ounces cottage cheese
1 scoop tuna	1 medium hamburger patty
1 cup lentil soup	8 ounces tofu
2 tablespoons peanut butter	4 ounces turkey
3 ounces cheese	1 medium chicken breast

Do not use individual amino acid supplements or the liquid "protein" supplements used by bodybuilders to get the protein you need.
If you use sources other than real food to get your recommended
amount of protein, you may create a severe imbalance of amino acids
in your system. An excess of one amino acid can throw off the balance
in your system. In fact, drinking a great deal of diet soda can do
this as well. Aspartame (NutraSweet) is made from the amino acid
phenylalanine. Use food to get the protein you need. You can use
liquid amino preparations such as Bragg's aminos, however, to flavor
your food. Made from soy, they contain a full range of amino acids.

You may ask how to reconcile this "prohibition" with the sugges-
tion that you sometimes use a power shake as an alternative to breakfast. What makes the power shake work with your food plan is that it
combines foods (milk, fruit and oatmeal) with protein powder (soy
and other proteins combined to create complete proteins). The power
shake is used as an alternative to skipping a meal.

Remember, I am trying to have you think about your relationship
to food. About planning your food, buying, preparing and eating it.
Eating a meal is very different from taking something to get by. You
will start to understand this the more you work with it.

What About Cholesterol?

While eggs are high in protein (13 grams each), you may feel nervous
about eating them because of their high cholesterol. You may have

been told to avoid them if your cholesterol count is high. It is true that coronary heart disease correlates to elevated levels of cholesterol in the blood. However, the evidence linking dietary cholesterol (which is found in the food we eat) with the presence of cholesterol in the blood is not so clearly demonstrated.

There is a lot of scientific literature available now about the role of sugar in the formation of cholesterol within the body. Some credible evidence suggests that having a high level of insulin (the hormone that is released when you eat a lot of sugar) has a far greater impact on the formation of body cholesterol than the number of eggs you eat. In fact, a large number of my clients have reported a significant drop in their cholesterol count after they have minimized their sugars for six months. If you consume a high level of sugar (including alcohol) and foods made with refined white flour, you will have a high level of insulin. In this case, I recommend avoiding foods high in dietary cholesterol, like red meat and egg yolks.

If you have a cholesterol problem, do some homework. Get as informed as you can about cholesterol. Learn about the different points of view on the best way to reduce your level. If you take medication to reduce your cholesterol, blood pressure or blood sugar, stay in touch with your doctor as you use this food plan. Have your levels checked regularly. All of these factors may change as you change the way you eat, and your medication may need to be adjusted.

A Protein That Raises Serotonin

Eating protein causes change to your brain chemistry. One of the amino acids found in protein is called tryptophan and is used to make serotonin, the brain chemical that gives you good impulse control and makes you feel mellow, at peace with the world. As we discussed earlier, if you are sugar sensitive, you most likely have a low level of serotonin. To raise this level, you will want to eat foods that are higher in tryptophan.

Below is a list of foods with their levels of tryptophan. You can choose the kind of protein that fits your lifestyle.

Protein Food	Serving	Level of Tryptophan (mg)
Chicken (white)	4 oz.	390
Pork loin	4 oz.	390
Cheddar cheese	1 cup	330
Ground beef	4 oz.	320
Tuna	4 oz.	320
Tempeh	4 oz.	310
Cottage cheese	1 cup	300
Tofu	4 oz.	280
Salmon	4 oz.	250
Soy protein powder	1 oz. (2 Tbs.)	220
Scrambled eggs	2	200
Spaghetti, whole wheat	2 cups cooked	190
Kidney beans	1 cup	180
Quinoa (a grain)	1 cup cooked	170
Almonds	.5 cup	170
Lentils	1 cup cooked	160
Milk	8 oz.	110
Soy milk	8 oz.	110
Yogurt	8 oz.	70

esha Food Processor

Use this list as a guideline to help choose proteins with more tryptophan as you create a food plan which works for you. Animal proteins are higher in amino acids (and therefore tryptophan) than foods like milk or almonds. If you are vegetarian, quinoa and soy will give you more than enough tryptophan.

Giving Tryptophan a Helping Hand

Okay, now you know what foods to eat to boost your tryptophan intake. But having tryptophan available for making serotonin requires more than simply eating foods that contain it. After you eat protein your body breaks it down into its different amino acids. These amino acids travel to the brain in your bloodstream, but they cannot immediately enter your brain cells because there is a blood-brain barrier that controls what gets into your brain cells at any given time.

There are far fewer tryptophan molecules than other amino acid molecules, so they lose out in the competition to cross the barrier. Think of tryptophan as a runt that gets left behind in the shuffle. This means that even if you eat protein with high levels of tryptophan, that alone won't do the trick. The runt needs help. Your body has a special way to help the runt get across the blood-brain barrier. When the body releases insulin, the insulin seeks out amino acids to use for building muscle. But insulin isn't interested in the runt. It want only the big guys, so it carries the other amino acids to other parts of the body where muscle can be found, leaving little tryptophan behind to hop across the blood-brain barrier and be put to use making serotonin. And more serotonin makes you feel better.

Think about this. If you're eating foods with lots of tryptophan, all you need is a hit of insulin so the tryptophan in your bloodstream can get into your brain to make more serotonin, right? Doesn't this mean you should be eating candy, which will cause more insulin to be released and clear the way for little tryptophan to get into the brain cells? Won't a little candy relieve your depression? Wouldn't you want to be eating lots of chocolate, ice cream and other sweets to raise your serotonin level?

As mentioned in Chapter 5, this has been recommended by a number of professionals in the last few years despite the fact that it creates tremendous problems for people who are sugar sensitive. "Alter your mood by timing your use of sweets," they say. "Raise serotonin by having jelly beans before you go to bed." "Eat chocolate." In fact, research shows that people who have low levels of serotonin, particularly women who crave carbohydrates, are actually unconsciously trying to self-medicate their depression by eating sweets, white bread and pasta.

But like other nutritional advice for people with normal body chemistries, the advice to eat chocolate is not good for people who are sugar sensitive. For you—and others with your special body chemistry—raising your insulin level by eating carbohydrates like jelly beans, chocolate or French bread creates even more trouble.

Foods like these can send the level of sugar in your blood sky-high and set you up for a huge crash. True, you will get more than enough insulin to help little tryptophan cross the blood-brain barrier, but you will also get that blood sugar spike and plunge. In addition, sweet foods will cause a big release of beta-endorphin and that will prime your brain to crave even more sugar. Remember, we are trying to quiet the priming.

But since all carbohydrates raise your level of insulin, there are other ways to get tryptophan into your brain cells to make serotonin without the harmful effects of jelly beans or French bread. We are trying for a gradual insulin response, not a blood sugar spike. What choices are there beyond jelly beans? The lowly potato to the rescue!

If you are eating protein at every meal, you are raising the level of amino acids, including tryptophan, in your blood. Mr. Tryptophan is

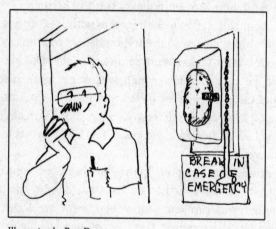

Illustration by Burt Dupre

waiting for his chance. Eating a baked potato before you go to bed raises the insulin level in the blood and moves the tryptophan to your brain. Your serotonin level rises in the middle of the night. This may even help you dream in a healthy way.

Does it have to be a potato? No, it can be any complex carbohydrate eaten without protein, like an apple, oatmeal (without milk or yogurt), a piece of toast or even orange juice. You could do it with a candy bar. But remember the *slower* the carbohydrate, the more effective the result.

Not only do potatoes give you a rise in insulin but they seem to offer emotional comfort as well. One scientific study (S. Holt et al., 1995) measured the "satiety index" of common foods. Satiety means feeling satisfied. This index gave a value to how well the foods gave the people eating them a sense of fullness. Here are a few of the foods they measured and the satiety rating they were given:

Food	Satiety Index
Potatoes	**323**
Wholemeal bread	157
Popcorn	154
Rice	138
Crackers	127
Cookies	120
Pasta	119
Cornflakes	118
Jelly beans	118
French fries	116
White bread	100
Ice cream	96
Chips	91
Doughnuts	68
Cake	65
Croissant	47

Mr. Spud is clearly the winner! Scientific investigation corroborated what all the sugar-sensitive people have been reporting. Eating potatoes is very satisfying. We'll talk in detail about this in the next chapter.

Protein Supplements

Some people have a very hard time eating breakfast. Or sometimes their work makes it impossible to get an evening meal. When you find it impossible to eat three meals a day, you can use a protein powder for one meal. Choose one which provides 20 to 28 grams of protein in a serving and fewer than 10 grams of sugars or carbohydrates. Most protein powders disguise sugars as complex carbohydrates. Read the labels.

We recommend this shake in our clinic as an occasional alternative to a meal:

George's Shake

- 1½ cups milk (preferably lactose-free), soy milk or oat milk

- ½ cup juice

- 2 tablespoons protein powder

- 2 tablespoons oatmeal (not "instant")

Put ingredients in the blender and blend on high for about a minute. If you do less, you will be crunching oats. Two tablespoons of protein powder will give you around 25 grams of protein, which is a good way to start the day. The oatmeal is a soluble fiber which provides a slow carbohydrate. This form of carbohydrate will give you energy for several hours. The milk is to provide the base for the drink. Using lactose-free milk will cut the sugars content of the milk. It is also easier to digest for some people. You can substitute the soy milk or oat milk if you don't eat dairy products. Sometimes soy milk is made with barley malt (a sugar) and will trigger sugar cravings. Also be cautious about using "rice" milk. It is very sweet and often seems to trigger cravings in sugar-sensitive people. Yes, the juice adds some sugar, but used in a small amount, it seems to be fine and people like the taste. Don't use only fruit juice in your drink (without any of the "milks"), though. More than ¹/₂ cup juice will provide too much sugar. Pay attention to your response to the ingredients. If you find yourself really, really liking any one of the ingredients, see what is going on. It's probably got too much sugar in it!

Remember, this shake should supplement your food plan, not replace it. Do not use a shake as an alternative to meals more than once a day. It is an option for hard times and should not be a regular substitute for eating real meals!

Settling into a Routine

Let yourself get stable with Step 4. Let eating three meals with protein become a habit. Spend two or three weeks feeling the effect of having increased your protein. Usually, increasing protein has a very positive impact. Continue to do your food journal so that you can observe the relationship between what you eat and how you feel. Eat three meals a day at regular intervals. Eat protein at each meal and maintain your vitamins. You are ready for Step 5.

Chapter 8

✱

Adjusting Your Carbohydrates

Congratulations! Now that you have completed Steps 1 through 4 and mastered having three meals with protein every day, you are ready for Step 5.

Step 5. Adjusting Your Carbohydrate Intake to Include More Complex Foods

In this step you start adjusting the kinds of carbohydrates you are eating. Carbohydrates include some alcoholic beverages (beer, wine and drinks mixed with fruit juice), sugars such as sucrose (table sugar), fructose (fruit sugar) and lactose (milk sugar), and starches like bread, pasta, cereal, vegetables, beans and grains.

Carbohydrates can be simple, like beer, wine and the sugars, or complex, like the starch found in brown rice or vegetables. Whether a carbohydrate is simple or complex depends on how many molecules it has. Sugars are considered simple carbohydrates, whereas starches are complex carbohydrates because they consist of three or more sugars joined together to make a long chain of molecules. Starches come from grains (wheat, corn, rice, etc.), beans (peas, lentils, chickpeas, etc.) and tubers (potatoes, yams, etc.).

Why do we care whether the carbohydrates we eat are simple or complex? Because in order for carbohydrates to be converted into fuel that your body can burn, their molecule chains must be short enough to go through the wall of your stomach or small intestine and get absorbed into your bloodstream. Before this can happen, your body has to digest the complex carbohydrates you have eaten, breaking them down into simpler forms. In fact, your body eventually breaks down all carbohydrates, even things like broccoli, into the simplest form of sugar, called glucose. When we talk about your blood sugar level what we are actually talking about is the amount of glucose in your blood. Remember that sugar is not bad. In fact, it is life-giving. But we want you to have all the positive effects of sugar in your body without the negative effects.

To prevent your sugar-sensitive body from getting too big a rush of sugar and sending your blood sugar skyrocketing (and later plummeting), you want to slow down the release of sugar into your bloodstream. You also want to avoid the beta-endorphin priming that comes with having alcohol or simple sugars. Avoiding simple carbohydrates, which are absorbed into your bloodstream quickly, and eating more complex carbohydrates, which are absorbed slowly, can help do this.

In addition, certain carbohydrates like whole grains and vegetables contain fibers that are difficult for your body to break down. Fibers are made from long chains of glucose that are joined together as either cellulose or pectin. Your body cannot digest cellulose fibers like bran, so they provide bulk but little nutritional value. Pectin fibers, such as apples, oats and beans, are water soluble and can be digested. Water-soluble fibers are great allies for sugar-sensitive people because the body takes longer to break down their long chains of molecules. The small intestine has to work hard to get the glucose out. This takes time and creates a stable, steady stream of sugar into the blood. For example, whole grain bread is "slower" than French bread because the brown part is the fiber.

The Carbohydrate Continuum

In Step 5 of your food plan you will start to shift your carbohydrate intake away from the quickly digested simple carbohydrates to the slower, more complex ones. You will eat fewer foods made with white flour and start eating more whole grains and foods with soluble fiber.

The carbohydrate continuum below shows the relative complexity of different carbohydrates. To the left are carbohydrates that are absorbed most quickly into your bloodstream. To the right are carbohydrates that contain a lot of soluble fiber and are absorbed more slowly.

This chart gives you general guidelines, but remember that a certain food may be slower or faster to break down depending upon how it's prepared. Digesting a baked potato with skin takes longer than digesting mashed potatoes because the brown skin of the potato contains fiber. Digesting cooked broccoli is faster than digesting raw

The Carbohydrate Continuum

Alcohol	Simple Sugars	Simple Starch	Complex Starches	Complex Starches	Wood
beer	glucose	**"white things"**	**"brown things"**	**"green things"**	not digestible
wine	sucrose	white-flour products	whole grains	broccoli and other green vegetables	
	fructose	white rice	beans		
	white sugar	pasta	potatoes	**"yellow things"**	
	honey		roots	squash and other yellow vegetables	
	corn syrup				
	all the others				

Your body eventually breaks all carbohydrates down to glucose. How quickly your body can do this depends on how complex the food is. The foods on the left of the continuum are very simple with only a few molecules. They are absorbed rapidly. The foods on the right of the continuum are very complex and require the body to work hard to break them down. This takes a long time and means that you will not get a sugar high from broccoli!

broccoli because the cooking breaks down the fiber before you eat it. Your body has to do less work.

When you design your food plan, you will want to include a good supply of complex carbohydrates. Choose the slowest ones. Learn to use the carbohydrate continuum. (A detailed edition can be found on the opposite page.) Start moving from "white things" to "brown" and "green" things on the carbohydrate continuum.

Now let's take a look at the continuum in more detail.

Alcohol

Alcohol is made by adding yeast to certain foodstuffs in order to ferment them. Wine is made by fermenting grapes or other fruits, beer by fermenting grain, and hard liquors by first fermenting grain and then distilling the ferment to make it more concentrated. So beer and wine contain a high level of fructose (a simple sugar) and alcohol, which can be absorbed directly from the stomach and requires no digestion at all. Hard liquor does not contain carbohydrate because it is a distillate of the carbohydrate base from which it is made. However, if it is mixed with fruit juice, it becomes even more potent for you. The result is that drinking alcoholic beverages is going to have a nearly immediate (and devastating) effect on your blood sugar level as well as cause beta-endorphin priming.

Simple Sugars

Sugars are found in an extraordinary variety of foods. Most of us recognize that candy bars, cake, cookies, sweetened cereals, chocolate milk, soda and ice cream contain sugars. But few people realize how many other foods contain hidden sugars. Canned ravioli, Slim-Fast, nutritional bars, prepared meatloaf dinners and dried fruit can contain more sugars than you might expect.

The list on the next page will give you a sense of how many foods contain overt sugar. Most people have no idea that sugar comes in so many forms. The sugars in bold print—overt sugars—are the ones that most people know about and use. Remember, though, that everything on this list is a sugar.

barley malt

beet sugar

brown rice syrup

brown sugar

cane juice

fruit juice
   concentrate

galactose

glucose

granulated sugar

high-fructose corn
   syrup

honey

invert sugar

lactose

**confectioners'
   sugar**

corn sweetener

corn syrup

date sugar

malted barley

maltodextrin

maltose

mannitol, sorbitol,
   xylitol, maltitol

maple sugar

microcrystalline
   cellulose

molasses

polydextrose

dextrin

dextrose

fructose

fructo-
   oligosaccharides

powdered sugar

raisin juice

raisin syrup

raw sugar

SUCANAT

sucrose

sugarcane

turbinado sugar

unrefined sugar

white sugar

I classify sugars as overt if they are obviously sugars and covert if they are hidden. Let's take a look at the sugar content of some of the foods you might be eating regularly, which I classify as overt sugar foods. I have calculated the "impact" value for each of these overt sugars by determining the density of the sugars and fiber in proportion to the total carbohydrate and then factoring in the portion size. The higher the impact number, the more intense the sugar hit. I have ranked them according to their impact value on the opposite page.

The typical "dose" of sugars in manufactured foods runs about 35 to 40 grams per serving. If you start to read labels, you will be surprised to see how consistent this level of sugar is. Observe your own response to the taste of sweet foods. Usually we have come to expect that this level of sugar tastes right. Sugar-sensitive people tend to be more comfortable with sweeter foods. Remember Dr. Kampov-Polevoy's experiments with alcoholic men who preferred drinks that were so much sweeter than the drinks preferred by nonalcoholics?

Food	Serving Size	Grams of Sugars	Impact
Ice cream Blizzard	1	88	72.08
M&M's	15 oz. package	82	64.04
McD's chocolate shake	16 oz.	58	53.16
ice cream	8 oz. (½ pint)	45	44.68
Coca-Cola	12 oz. can	39	39.02
Kool-Aid	12 oz.	38	37.50
chocolate chips	½ cup	43	33.25
chocolate cake with icing	1 piece	31	26.31
frozen yogurt, soft serve	1 cup	32	24.38
Butterfinger candy	2.16 oz.	30	20.97
Jell-O pudding snack	1	23	18.89
maple syrup	3 oz.	30	18.39
chocolate milk	8 oz.	20	15.72
Jell-O snack	1	18	18.00
white sugar	2 packets	16	11.99
gum	1 stick	2	.67

esha Food Processor. Impact score by DesMaisons

Fruits and fruit juices are also high in sugars. Most people assume that the sugars found in fruit are very healthy because they are natural. It is true that fruits contain vitamins not found in products like Coca-Cola. However, your sugar-sensitive body registers the sugar in fruit and responds to it as powerfully as to the sugar in chocolate chips. Fruit juice in particular is a sugar with a high impact because it has very little fiber to slow it down. Let's take a look at the sugar content of some fruit juices on the next page.

Although drinking orange juice instead of cola is more nutritious, the sugar content is almost exactly the same. Also, notice how much more sugar grape juice contains. This is why concentrated grape juice is so often used as a sweetener in "natural" foods. People think that grape juice is healthier than refined white sugar. But your response to a certain food is determined by the intensity of the sugar hit.

12 oz. Juice	Grams of Sugar
grape	54
apple	41
orange	38
grapefruit	27
tomato	8

esha Food Processor

Let's take a look now at the sugar in whole fruits:

Food	Serving Size	Grams of Carbs	Grams of Sugars	Grams of Fiber	Impact
applesauce, sweetened	1 cup	50.75	47.66	3.06	41.89
raisins	1 box (1.5 oz.)	34.01	32.29	1.72	29.03
grapes	1 cup	24.48	27.52	1.60	25.05
dried apricots	½ cup	50.22	33.44	4.18	19.48
apple with peel	1 large	32.44	25.44	5.72	15.46
banana	1 medium	27.61	21.82	2.83	15.00
orange	1 large	21.71	17.30	4.42	10.26
pear	1 medium	25.07	17.50	3.98	9.43
blueberries	½ cup	10.22	8.27	1.96	5.10
strawberries	½ cup	5.05	4.06	1.66	1.93
apricots	1	3.89	3.05	.84	1.73
raspberries	½ cup	7.13	5.84	4.18	1.36

esha Food Processor. Impact score by DesMaisons

Compare the impact values of these to those in the chart for overt sugars. You will start to see why making some small changes can have a huge effect on how you feel. These charts will show you how to identify the overt sugars in your diet. Start noticing how often you have sugar foods. Mark them in your food journal. Don't get discouraged if you find that a significant proportion of what you eat is high in sugar.

Don't stop eating sugar foods yet, but start being attentive. If you have something sweet, plan to have it with your meals so that you temper the impact of the sugar with the other foods you are eating. Start cutting down on the overts as best you can. But don't scare yourself. Remember, this plan is not about deprivation. It's about paying attention and making informed choices. The more you understand how all of this fits together and the more you understand the equation of your own body, the better you will be able to make choices that work for you.

Think about ways you can creatively have sweet foods that you like. Have whole fruit (with fiber) instead of juice. Substitute juice for soda because it is more nutritious, but dilute the juice so you won't get a huge sugar hit. For example, if you make a juice spritzer with 3 ounces of orange juice and 9 ounces of sparkling water instead of having a can of soda, you can reduce your sugar intake drastically. If you have been drinking four sodas a day, you will cut your daily sugar intake by 112 grams!

My clients frequently ask me about the advisability of using "sugar-free" products. There are two parts to the answer. Many products advertised as "sugar-free" are free from certain kinds of sugars. If a manufacturer uses a trisaccharide (a sugar with three parts in it), it does not have to be called a sugar since legally it is a starch. Maltodextrin falls into this category, and you will respond to it as if it were a sugar.

Other sugar-free products use aspartame (NutraSweet) as a sweetener. Aspartame is made from phenylalanine, which is an amino acid. High doses of any single amino acid can throw off the balance of aminos in your brain and body. Since phenylalanine is a precursor to dopamine and norepinephrine, which are both stimulating neurotransmitters, high usage of NutraSweet can create an "upper"-like effect. You may find that you really like the effect you get from sugar-free products. I encourage my clients to stay away from products with aspartame both for their addictive potential and their reinforcement of the dependence upon sweet taste. I will talk more about aspartame on p. 146.

Many people have switched from ice cream to low-fat frozen yogurt as a way to reduce calories. Low-fat yogurt has fewer calories from fat but far more from sugar. A sugar-sensitive person does better with real ice cream because the fat it contains actually slows the speed at which the sugar is absorbed into your bloodstream. Now, I am not advocating the long-term use of ice cream, but if you do eat these desserts, you might experiment to see whether ice cream or fat-free frozen yogurt affects you differently.

Your goal right now is to notice the sugars in your diet and to start reducing your consumption of overt sugars.

"White Things"

The carbohydrate continuum chart will help you see the relationship between sugar and what I call white things, brown things and green things. I use these terms because it is easy to remember these simple images as you make your own food choices. Just as you have begun to notice the sugars, I now want you to look at the simple starches in your diet. I use the term "white things" to identify refined starches. The term is apt because they have literally had the brown part of the grain removed to make them more visually attractive. Taking out the brown part also makes them sweeter because it takes less time for your body to digest the starch and convert it to sugar.

Here are some examples of "white things":

bagels	noodles
cake	pancakes made with white flour
cereal	pasta
cookies	pastry
crackers	pie
croissants	pita bread
doughnuts	risotto
English muffins	spaghetti
flour tortillas	waffles
macaroni	white bread
muffins	white rice

The chart that follows shows you the amounts of carbohydrate, sugar and fiber, and also includes the impact value. It gives you a clear sense of how the level of fiber can slow the impact of the sugars.

A Comparison of "White Things"

White Thing	Serving Size	Grams of Carbs	Grams of Sugar	Grams of Fiber	Impact
doughnut, powdered sugar	1	24.0	12.0	1.0	5.5
cornbread (KFC)	1	25.0	10.0	1.0	3.6
raisin bran cereal (Kellogg's)	1 cup	42.9	15.0	7.0	2.7
plain pancakes (4" each)	3	41.8	10.0	9.0	1.8
blueberry muffin	1	27.3	6.0	1.0	0.88
Rice Krispies cereal (Kellogg's)	1 cup	22.8	2.0	0.3	0.21
bread (firm white)	1 slice	33.2	3.0	1.5	0.08
cornflakes cereal (Kellogg's)	1 cup	21.6	2.0	0.7	0.08
bread (soft white)	1 slice	28.6	2.2	1.2	0.08
English muffin	2	52.0	3.9	3.0	0.07
crackers (Ritz)	8	14.6	1.2	.38	0.07
croissant	1	26.1	1.8	1.5	0.03
white rice (cooked)	1 cup	44.6	0.32	0.63	0.00
crackers (saltines)	8	17.2	0.36	0.72	—.01
pita bread (6½" diameter)	1	33.4	0.78	1.32	—.01
bagel	1	37.9	1.07	1.63	—.02
flour tortillas (10" round)	1	40.3	0.87	2.38	—.03
spaghetti (cooked)	2 cups	79.2	3.64	7.56	—.18

esha Food Processor. Impact score by DesMaisons

Compare the impact values to the items in the overt sugar list as well.

These are considered typical servings in the nutrition tables. You may eat a larger slice of pie than 2 inches or more than ½ cup of rice. Adjust the comparisons according to the size of the serving you eat. If you have 2 cups of raisin bran cereal for breakfast, you will have more than twice the sugar in a sugar doughnut. You will start to see why it is important to read labels.

You may look at this chart and say, "Well, now, which is the best white thing for me to eat?" And you can see that a bagel is better than white bread because it has a little more fiber. But wait before choosing the "best" white thing. Look at the "brown things" list which follows and you will begin to see the dramatic difference between white and brown things.

Most commercially sold bread contains refined white flour even though it is labeled as brown or whole grain. For example, breads with wheat flour or flour at the head of their ingredients lists are still made with refined white flour. Unless the first ingredient is whole wheat flour, think of it as a white thing.

Also check the food label for the amount of fiber. Look for 2 or more grams of fiber in each serving. You can see that white things are white because they don't have much fiber. Remember, the higher the fiber, the longer it will take to digest and the slower the flow of sugar into your bloodstream will be.

Look at the fiber values for white things and compare them to the fiber in the chart of "brown things" on page 131. There is a big difference. Also remember that whole grains have far more nutritional value because the "brown stuff" has the vitamins in it. Take a page in your food journal now to make a list of the things you eat that have white flour in them. Your goal is to shift your intake of white things to brown things. For many of these foods, you can substitute whole grain products such as 100 percent whole wheat bread or whole wheat pasta.

You can have brown rice instead of white rice. You can try shredded wheat instead of Rice Krispies. Or you can have oatmeal, which is the best of all because so much of its fiber is soluble. Whole grain foods are more complex and give your body a solid, consistent fuel to draw from.

Cereal Choices

All-Bran (Kellogg's)	− 3.08
Oatmeal	− 0.11
Grape-Nuts	− 0.06
Cheerios	− 0.05
Shredded Wheat	0.00
Corn Flakes (Kellogg's)	0.08
Rice Krispies	0.20
Raisin Bran	2.67
Oatmeal (cinnamon/spice package)	5.70
Cap'n Crunch	6.19
Frosted Flakes	6.50

Impact score by DesMaisons

When you first looked at the list of white things, were you surprised to see how many of the foods you love were in that column? Sugar-sensitive people *love* white things—sometimes even more than ice cream or other sweet treats. It might spook you to think of not eating white things. Some people love breads more than anything. If so, be gentle with yourself. No one is going to take away your favorite foods. The idea is for you to move toward using more complex carbohydrates *as you can*. Maybe you can start by finding a new bread that is a little heartier than the one you eat now. Check out the cereal options. Be careful to read labels, though. Often foods that are labeled all natural and look brown are filled with sugars. Commercially made granola is often like this. It sure looks good for you, but it has grams and grams of sugar.

If you find that giving up white things is difficult, do what you have done with the sugars. Try not to eat them alone. Have your white thing with some other slow food. Make change at the pace that works for you. You do not have to hurry this process. We are looking for solid long-term success, not dramatic short-term results.

When you do eat from the "brown" and "green" side of the carbohydrate continuum rather than the "white" side, you'll start noticing big changes in your sense of well-being and your energy level. When you look at your food journal you will see the connection between your new way of eating and your feelings.

You may find that this step is hard. We love white things. They often represent comfort and love. Many people would kill for French bread. Notice your own emotional attachment to white things. See if you can tease out what part of your enjoyment of white things comes from the biochemical response they give you and what part of your enjoyment comes from your emotional association with what you are eating.

For example, for me sugar cookies in the shape of Christmas trees covered in green icing (or even plain) have a huge association with the joy of Christmas time. I found it very hard to even think about not eating them then. The idea of giving them up, even if I was pondering it in July, made me so sad and angry about having such a stupid body chemistry that I would go eat something sweet to comfort myself!

I had to learn to be patient with myself and understand the full emotional impact of those cookies. I found that the real feelings were about being cared for at Christmas. It seemed as if all the other children had mothers who made them cookies at Christmas. My mother worked so we rarely got those cookies. When my children were little, I started making them iced green Christmas tree cookies as a way to show them the love I had wanted when I was little. Once I realized this, I gave myself permission to have some cookies at Christmas, but I also paid attention to the bigger picture of all the white things that are associated with holidays and showing love. I chose to eat a few cookies because that seemed the most important emotionally. But I didn't eat the pies and the cakes and the sweet breads. I learned to recognize the many emotional issues wrapped up in the foods I wanted and made choices that would support my food plan. Now I don't even crave the Christmas tree cookies. (But I still make them and give them to my friends who aren't sugar sensitive.)

The bottom line is, do what you can to shift your carbohydrate intake from white things to brown things. But do it at the rate you feel comfortable with.

"Brown Things"

"Brown things" include the foods higher in fiber, such as whole grains, seeds and beans. This list shows examples of what I call brown things.

amaranth
black beans
brown rice
cornmeal
garbanzo beans
   (chickpeas)
granola, no sugar added
hummus
kidney beans (used in
   chili)
lentils
millet
oat bran
oatmeal
pasta (whole wheat)
polenta
popcorn

potatoes with skin
pumpkin seeds
quinoa
refried beans
soy beans
sunflower seeds
sweet potato
whole grain bread
whole grain cereal
whole grain pancakes
whole grain pasta
whole grain tortillas
   (corn or
   whole wheat)
whole wheat flour
yams

Brown things are an excellent source of complex carbohydrates. You might recognize some of these foods from the protein chart. Beans and grains contain both protein and carbohydrate. Grains can have 24 percent of their cooked weight as carbohydrate and 3 percent as protein while beans can have 19 percent of their weight as carbohydrate and 8 percent as protein. Brown things provide your body with solid nourishment and sustained energy. They will help you maintain a steady blood sugar level and support the optimal-level feelings we talked about in Chapter 3. Here again is the chart showing the difference in your feelings between times when your blood sugar is at an optimal level and when it has plummeted as a result of eating sugars and foods made with refined flour. These are just a few of the many benefits of switching from white things to brown things.

Optimal Blood Sugar	Low Blood Sugar
Energetic	Tired all the time
Tired when appropriate	Tired for no reason
Focused and relaxed	Restless, can't keep still
Clear	Confused
Having a good memory	Having trouble remembering
Able to concentrate	Having trouble concentrating
Able to solve problems effectively	Easily frustrated
Easygoing	More irritable than usual
Even-tempered	Getting angry unexpectedly

The next chart will show you the sugar and fiber content and the impact score of various brown things. All servings in this chart reflect 1/2 cup of cooked (in this case, boiled) food. Compare the grams of fiber to those listed in the "white things" chart. Notice how many have more than 2 grams of fiber. Adjust the fiber and other values according to how much you usually eat.

Compare the foods in this chart to those on the "white things" list. The higher levels of fiber in the brown things are what slow the sugar absorption down and keep your blood sugar and brain chemicals at optimal levels.

As you add brown things to your diet, keep noticing how you respond to what you are eating. If you find yourself becoming really attached to a given food, try to sort out what is going on. Anne Marie developed a recipe for a pumpkin pudding she could eat for breakfast. It seemed like a good idea—it was a brown thing and had no sugar in it. However, over a couple of months of working together on her food plan, we noticed that she was becoming more and more attached to her pudding. Breakfast was important because she could have the pudding. If she skipped it for another food, she would spend the day thinking about the pudding. I really wasn't sure why this was happening, but I suggested to Anne Marie that the pumpkin pudding seemed to be acting as a trigger food and she might want to substitute something else. She agreed and changed her breakfast.

A Comparison of "Brown Things"

Brown Thing	Serving Size	Grams of Carbs	Grams of Sugar	Grams of Fiber	Impact
popcorn	1 cup	6.23	0.00	1.21	.00
hummus	½ cup	24.80	0.00	6.27	.00
refried beans	½ cup	23.30	0.00	6.00	.00
peanuts	½ cup	15.70	0.00	5.80	.00
brown rice	1 cup	44.80	3.20	3.51	−.03
sweet potato	1 medium	27.70	1.54	3.08	−.09
baked potato with skin	1 medium	50.90	3.64	4.85	−.09
whole grain bread	2 slices	25.80	3.01	3.80	−.10
oatmeal (cooked)	1 cup	25.20	1.64	3.98	−.15
pasta (whole wheat), cooked	2 cups	74.20	10.90	12.60	−.25
quinoa	1 cup	104.20	14.11	15.98	−.25
garbanzo beans, cooked	½ cup	22.40	4.30	6.30	−.37
kidney beans	½ cup	20.80	3.35	5.66	−.38
soy beans, cooked	½ cup	8.50	4.30	5.60	−.50
almonds	½ cup	16.70	8.41	9.45	−.52
black beans, cooked	½ cup	20.40	5.42	7.48	−.55
lentils, cooked	½ cup	19.90	7.72	9.21	−.58

esha Food Processor. Impact score by DesMaisons

I have seen this same sort of unexpected response in my clients to several different things on the brown list like sunflower seeds or corn products. Your job is to pay attention and notice whether any food, be it white, brown, green or yellow, is hooking you. A major part of the work you are doing with this food plan is to move away from an addictive relationship to what you eat. Each person has a different response to these foods. If the food makes you crazy, sort out what is going on. Use your food journal to figure it out. Experiment. Look at the different pieces. Try new alternatives.

"Green Things"

Green things are vegetables. They are a valuable part of your food plan because they are slow carbohydrates and provide lots of vitamins and minerals as well. Try to eat lots of green things. (Actually, some of your green things will be yellow, orange, red or white—like carrots, red peppers and radishes—instead of green, but saying green things is shorter.) Vegetables are complex carbohydrates that have long chains of molecules and plenty of fiber, which make them slow to digest. Try to eat vegetables at both lunch and dinner. Make salad regularly. Raw vegetables are slower to digest than cooked ones; cooking vegetables breaks down their fiber instead of letting your stomach do it.

Some people who are sugar sensitive have had little experience with vegetables. If this is true for you, pick the vegetables which seem the most familiar and start with those. If preparing fresh vegetables makes you nervous, start with frozen ones. They are easy and quick to make, as well as tasty.

Here is a list of the kinds of vegetables I eat:

asparagus	Chinese cabbage	lima beans
avocados	corn	mushrooms
bean sprouts	cucumbers	okra
beets	eggplant	onions
broccoli	garlic	parsnips
Brussels sprouts	green beans and	peas
cabbage (white and	wax beans	radishes
red)	green, red and	spinach
carrots	yellow peppers	squash
cauliflower	jicama	tomatoes
celery	kale	zucchini
chili peppers	lettuce	

The next chart shows you the relative amount of fiber in some of these vegetables. The higher the ratio of fiber to total carbohydrate, the slower the carbohydrate is digested. Take a look at the listing for Brussels sprouts. Do you see that almost half of the carbohydrate in Brussels sprouts is fiber? That makes them a very slow green thing. And that's exactly why green and brown things are a better option for you than white things. It's also why we never get high from broccoli and its cousins. Have you ever heard of anyone who would kill for Brussels sprouts? For pasta maybe, but not for Brussels sprouts! While searching through Medline, I found a scientific article about the "addictive" characteristics of carrots. It reported that one subject had an unusually strong attachment to them. Carrots have more sugars relative to many other vegetables, although certainly nothing like the sugars in white things. But pay attention. If you start hoarding your own stash of carrots, you may be on to something.

A Comparison of "Green Things"

Vegetable	Serving Size	Grams of Carbs	Grams of Sugar	Grams of Fiber	Impact
carrots (7.5")	1	7.27	4.75	2.16	1.69
tomato	1 medium	5.71	3.44	1.35	1.26
pepper, green bell	1 medium	4.76	1.85	1.33	.20
lettuce, iceberg	1 cup	1.15	0.88	.77	.08
green peas	1 cup	22.88	8.80	8.80	0.00
asparagus spears	6	3.81	1.44	1.44	0.00
spinach (cooked)	1 cup	10.15	0.00	6.84	0.00
corn	1 cup	32.14	2.95	4.43	− 0.14
green beans	1 cup	8.71	3.51	4.05	− 0.22
cabbage	1 cup	6.69	2.51	3.45	− 0.35
Brussels sprouts	1 cup	12.90	5.32	6.36	− 0.43
veggies, frozen	1 cup	23.84	5.82	8.01	− 0.53
broccoli	1 cup	9.84	3.31	5.52	− 0.74
lima beans	1 cup	35.10	5.04	10.60	− 0.83

esha Food Processor. Impact score by DesMaisons

Fruit

Now that you have a bigger picture of carbohydrates, let's go back to the fruit story. Earlier in this chapter we saw that fruits have a fair amount of sugar. But, like brown things and green things, the impact of the sugar in fruits is tempered by the fiber they contain. The amount of fiber in the fruit affects where the fruit falls on the carbohydrate continuum. For example, raisins would fall near the left end as very, very sweet, while raspberries might fall closer to broccoli. These differences make it difficult to include fruit in the carbohydrate continuum. Here is a separate continuum showing only fruits, so you can see how they compare with one another in terms of sugar and fiber. I generally spend a lot of time talking about fruits with my clients. Fruits become an important part of your recovery as you start to take overt sugars out of your diet. It is far too easy to slip into substituting a lot of fruit for the sugars you are trying to remove. Learn the differences in the fruit values.

Look back at your food journal and see if you can discern what effect fruit has on you. Which fruits are you most drawn to? Do you like raspberries or raisins more? Look at the fiber ratios for each. Raspberries have a lot of fiber so the sugar hit is minimal. Raisins, on the other hand, have no fiber and their carbohydrate is almost entirely sugar. This is why sugar-sensitive people usually prefer raisins to raspberries.

Remember what happens when you turn a whole fruit into a juice. The fiber ratio goes down because there is less fiber to slow the sugar down. The same thing happens when you cook the fruit. Look at the difference between applesauce and apples.

Remember to consider the impact of drying fruit. Drying fruit removes the water and makes the sugar far denser. A 1/2 cup of raisins has 63 grams of sugar, while a Coke has "only" 38, a candy bar "only" 40. You might snack on six pieces of dried banana even though you would never eat three whole bananas at one time. Don't be misled by the "small" portions of dried fruit. Think of them as concentrated sugar!

The Fruit Continuum

Most Impact			Moderate Impact		Least Impact
50	40	30	20	10	0
Raisins (58)	Applesauce, sweetened (42)	Orange juice (36)	Figs (20)	Cherries (11)	Peach (5)
Grape juice (55)	Apple juice (39)	Prune juice (34)	Dried apricots (19)	Oranges (10)	Blueberries (5)
Cranberry juice cocktail (53)		Grapes (25)	Applesauce, unsweetened (18)	Cantaloupe (10)	Plums (4)
Pineapple juice (50)			Apple, large (15)	Watermelon (9)	Strawberries (2)
			Banana (15)		Apricot, fresh (2)
			Pineapple (14)		Raspberries (1)

Serving Sizes: raisins (3 oz.); grape juice (12 fl. oz.); cranberry juice cocktail (12 fl. oz.); pineapple juice (12 fl. oz.); applesauce, sweetened (1 cup); apple juice (12 fl. oz.); orange juice (12 fl. oz.); prune juice (12 fl. oz.); grapes (1 cup); dried figs (4); dried apricots (½ cup); applesauce, unsweetened (1 cup); apple (large); banana (medium); pineapple (fresh, 1 cup); cherries (15); orange (large); cantaloupe (1 cup); watermelon (1 cup); peach (medium); blueberries (½ cup); plum (medium); strawberries (½ cup); apricot (1); raspberries (½ cup)

Shifting Your Place on the Continuum

As you work with these charts, you can begin to get a sense of where you are on the carbohydrate continuum. Work at moving your eating from the left and simple side to the right and more complex side. Experiment with your food plan to introduce little changes which support the shift. Be gentle and patient with yourself. Factor in the emotional attachment you may have to sugars or white things. Take things as slowly as you are comfortable with. And really praise yourself for whatever steps you are making in moving to the green side of the carbohydrate continuum.

Chapter 9

✦

Sugars and You

In doing the first five steps, you have created a solid foundation for your recovery from the problems caused by sugar sensitivity. You have been working hard to eat in a stable and consistent way. You have started to shift your place on the carbohydrate continuum toward eating more whole grains and less white flour and sugar. You are still keeping your food journal. These tools have served you well and will continue to do so. Let's check in with where we are with the program.

---

1. Keeping a food journal

2. Eating three meals a day at regular intervals

3. Taking vitamins as recommended

4. Eating the recommended amount of protein at each meal

5. Adjusting your carbohydrate intake to include more complex foods

6. **Reducing or eliminating sugars (including alcohol)**

7. Creating a plan for maintenance

Now you are ready to begin directly addressing the foods that create problems for you. From the healing you have achieved, you will be ready to let go of the things which have caused so much trouble.

Step 6: Reducing or Eliminating Sugars

In this step, you will continue the pattern of creating biochemical stability with each food and lifestyle change, and begin to proceed to the more difficult transitions. This will ensure that your food plan is safe, effective and long-term. As you do Step 6, reducing or eliminating sugars, you will understand why I have been so insistent about taking only one step at a time. Had you tried to go off sugars your first week, you would have felt terrible. But when you do Step 6 after achieving the first five steps, your recovery from the compulsive use of alcohol, sugars and foods made with refined white flour can be a progressive and successful process.

On the Trail of Secret Sugars

Now that you have a better sense of the overt sugars, let's go back to the covert sugars. Look at your food journal. Use a different colored marker and identify all the kinds of sugars you eat. Start with the overt sugars, then mark all the other foods in which you think sugar is found. In how many places do you find sugars? Low-fat products often hide the most sugar. When food manufacturers take out the fat, guess what they use to replace the taste factor?

Also, take a close look at foods that proclaim "no sugar." Remember that "no sugar" simply means "no sucrose." Manufacturers use different kinds of sweeteners to mask how much sugar is in products marketed as "healthy" or "low-fat." The labels on these foods may show five different ingredients, such as maltodextrin, raisin juice or fructose. These all sound healthy, don't they? They are all sugars. Your taste buds and body will recognize them as sugars even though the label may say "sugar-free." Read the labels carefully. The new labeling requirements demand that the manufacturer show both the "carbohydrate" and the "sugar" content. However, how the manufacturer defines the sugar may differ somewhat from what we would call a sugar. For example, brown rice syrup can legally be called only a carbohydrate because it is made from rice, which is a starch, not a sugar. So you will have to use your judgment in this process.

One power bar sold at the gym for bodybuilding has *twelve* different kinds of sugars. Of course, eating one of these would make you feel wonderful in the short run because it would spike your blood sugar level and give you a beta-endorphin hit. But you now realize that what first feels like a positive effect is hardly that for you. This kind of power bar will not affect your serotonin level the way a candy bar might. Can you figure out why? The power bars also have protein in them. If you have something sweet combined with the protein you will not get a rise in tryptophan because the new aminos in the protein will still compete with little runt tryptophan. Eating sweets and protein together will not give you the serotonin effect.

Eating protein at the same time you have something sweet *will* slow down the effect on your blood sugar level. When you eat more complex foods with simple ones, the digestion of the simple ones takes longer. This is why having alcohol with a meal creates less of an effect than having it without food. Let's look at an example.

Ron was doing serious bodybuilding, but he couldn't understand why his training program wasn't giving him the results he wanted. He drank gallons of Gatorade at the gym. He used "weight gain" muscle powder daily. He sincerely believed he was eating a very healthy diet. Ron recently had decided to "balance" his nutrition program and added a new meal-replacement bar. He thought he was doing everything right, but his weight and muscle development wouldn't budge. I had him bring in the ingredient labels from the meal-replacement bars and the muscle powder. We read them together and wrote down the names of the sugars they contained. There were *nineteen* different forms of sugar in these two products. "Balanced" or not, these products didn't work for Ron. He was sugar sensitive.

Then Ron changed his nutrition plan to include more real food rather than the bodybuilding supplement products. He started eating three meals, increased his food protein, replaced "white things" with whole grain products and took out most of the sugars from his diet. His energy . increased immediately and his endurance escalated. Within three weeks he began seeing the results in his muscle development and workout plan. What Ron had worked so hard for unsuccessfully during the past year finally started happening.

You can start the way Ron did. Read the label before you eat a food. Look at grams of sugar. It may help to visually translate grams into teaspoons. Four grams equals 1 teaspoon of sugar. If a 12-ounce can of soda has 39 grams of sugar, that means you are drinking nearly 10 teaspoons of sugar with each can. If you put 10 teaspoons of sugar on a plate and look at how much it is, you may find it easier to cut down.

The infamous "nutrition" bar says "no high-fructose corn syrup" and "low fat" on the label. The ingredients include rolled oats, *brown rice syrup* and/or FruitSource (whole *rice syrup* and *grape juice concentrate*), rice flour, oat bran, *pear juice concentrate*, cornmeal, *figs*, *barley malt*, cocoa powder, rice crisp, *chocolate chips*, coffee beans, natural flavors and leavening. The label says it has 52 grams of carbohydrate, 2 grams of fiber and 16 grams of sugars. It isn't quite clear which are the sugars and which are the carbs. But the brown rice syrup, figs and barley malt may be classed as carbohydrates rather than sugar. Your body will respond to them as sugars.

Notice that the ingredients are listed in the order of the amounts (this is true of *all* ingredient lists on packaged foods). By using seven different sugars and carbohydrates, the manufacturer keeps you from easily seeing that the bar is mainly sugar and oats. But the large print on the label is designed to convince you what a healthy alternative this is.

Take It Easy

You may be overwhelmed when you see all the places sugars are hidden. Manufacturers like to add sugar. It makes products taste "better" so more people will buy them. After you have looked at a number of labels, you may wonder what you will be able to eat if you decide to eliminate sugars. Or you may have a powerful emotional response that life without sugar just isn't worth the effort. Don't scare yourself.

You are just learning to read labels. Be gentle with yourself. You aren't going to take out every single sugar from your diet. You will develop good detective skills so you know where sugar lurks. This awareness will let you move from an unconscious attachment to sweets toward a conscious choice about what you eat. If you know that a can of soda has 10 teaspoons of sugar, you can choose to have it or not. Conscious awareness will give you the opportunity to measure the impact. You can choose your trade-offs. You may find that it is not such a big deal to have 3 ounces of orange juice in sparkling water rather than soda because you feel so much better. You may find that more and more you like reducing the amount of sugars you eat.

A Guide to the Sugar Content of Some "Diet" Foods

As you have been working on shifting your place on the carbohydrate continuum, you have already started looking at sugars in different foods. Let's look at some of the sugars in foods you might not have identified as sugar foods yet.

This chart includes foods that you might not have thought of as sources of sugar. Who would think Ensure and Slim-Fast would have more sugar than a soda? Or that Instant Breakfast is 100 percent sugar? Doing Step 6 of your food plan will demand shifting the way you think about what you eat. If you have been diligently keeping to

Type of Food	Serving Size	Grams of Carbohydrate	Grams of Sugar
diet drink (Ultra Slim-Fast)	12 oz.	48	36
Instant Breakfast	1 package	28	28
Chocolate drink (Ensure)	8 oz.	47	22
apple bran muffin (McDonald's)	1	40	21
Fruit Leather	1 roll	17	9

esha Food Processor. Impact score by DesMaisons

a low-fat regime, you may feel cheated to have to give up sugar, too. So as you take out the sugar in your diet, you will probably increase the fat a little. Just as you shouldn't substitute sugar for fat, do not substitute fat for sugar. The name of the game is paying attention, knowing what you are eating and noticing the effect it has on your moods and your body.

The Next Step

After you have worked at shifting to the more complex side of the carbohydrate continuum and reducing your sugars, you may decide that you are ready to go ahead and eliminate overt sugars altogether. If you feel you are ready to do this, start by thinking of it as a detox process. You will be giving up your "drug" and will want to plan a way to minimize your discomfort and maximize your success. Thinking of going off sugar as detox will also help you see that there will be predictable physiological stages and, most important, light at the other end of the tunnel. Going off sugars doesn't have to be too difficult from a physical standpoint. It may be more difficult from an emotional standpoint. But we will talk about this as we go.

There is a *huge* payoff if you choose to eliminate most sugars from your diet. You will feel better than you ever have. You will still get the "good" feelings sugar has given you—the increase in serotonin and beta-endorphin—but you will get these in a new way. The skills you have developed as a food chemist and meal planner will work in your service. You will intentionally create your own good feelings with your food choices. You will like this new state a lot.

In getting ready for sugar detox, you will want to look at your alcohol use. Since you will remember that alcoholic beverages are the quickest sugars, they will be included in your sugar detox plan. But if you are biochemically dependent upon alcohol, you will experience alcohol withdrawal when you stop drinking. I want you to stay safe in the process.

Since you may not know if you have a problem with alcohol, let's take a look at a quick assessment tool to help you sort this out. Answer these four questions:

Have you ever felt you should cut down on your drinking?
Have people ever annoyed you by criticizing your drinking?
Have you ever felt bad or guilty about your drinking?
Have you ever had a drink first thing in the morning (an eye-opener) to steady your nerves or to get rid of a hangover?

Give yourself one point for every yes answer you gave. If you have answered yes to any of these questions, you may have a problem with alcohol. Read the appendix on alcohol detox (page 209) before you eliminate alcohol from your diet.

Going Off Sugars

If you do not have a problem with alcohol, or if you have had a problem in the past and are now in recovery, and are ready to go off other sugars, go back to your food journal. This old friend will serve as your guide once again. Highlight the overt sugars you have been eating. Get a sense of what things you want to exclude from your diet. Decide whether you are going to first cut down and then cut out or whether you are going to go cold turkey. Neither way is better. What counts most is your style, how you like to make changes in your life. Draw from the experience you have had over the past few weeks in getting to know your own style. Do you take a gradual approach or do you plunge right in? Whichever way fits for you, use it when you create your food plan around reducing or eliminating sugars.

Most of my clients have found it easiest to cut down first as part of shifting their place on the carbohydrate continuum and then to pick a time to simply go cold turkey and eliminate the sugars that are left in their diets. You should choose what works for you.

Planning Your Sugar Detox

Withdrawal from sugar will feel like withdrawal from a drug. This is because both sugar and narcotics raise our beta-endorphin level, and when we stop using them the brain starts begging for more. Remember, as we saw in Chapter 5, sugar evokes a beta-endorphin response like an opiate drug such as morphine or heroin. Your withdrawal symptoms will certainly not be as severe as those of a heroin addict, but you too are "kicking the habit." You may get the shakes, feel nauseous and edgy or have diarrhea or headaches for a few days. You may be surprised by the intensity of the physical changes you feel.

If you do not have any physical symptoms when you go off sugar, there are several possibilities: you didn't use a lot of sugars to begin with, you are not sugar sensitive after all, or you are getting enough covert sugar that your brain doesn't notice any change.

Plan your sugar detox for a time when you do not have severe stress. The process usually takes five days, with the fourth day being the hardest. Think through the timing of your detox. Schedule it so that on the fourth day you have time to yourself. Do not start your detox so that the fourth day lands on the day you have to make a presentation to your major account. Do not plan the fourth day to coincide with your son's wedding. Be strategic.

Also, let the people around you know what you are doing. If your coworker has a huge bowl of M&M's on her desk, ask her if she might put them away while you go off sugar. Plan to stay away from the places that will trigger you. Don't go into the local coffee shop even for just coffee until you are well through your detox. The sight or smell of the sweet rolls may trigger your craving for your favorite sweet foods. I have been off sugar for many years, but I still cannot go into a Dunkin' Donuts without vividly recalling the old days when I always had two chocolate doughnuts with my coffee.

Plan to keep your other food intake as steady as possible and don't forget to use your food journal. Tell people ahead of time that you are going off sugar and will be going through a detox period. Get their support. Ask them to put away the bowls of candy if they can. This is a big step for you. If you lay the groundwork, going off sugar will not be as difficult as you might imagine and you will feel fabulous when you are done.

Doing It

Your withdrawal symptoms will be minimized and you will have very few cravings if you pay special attention to your food during your detox from sugar. Drink lots and lots of water. Fill a liter bottle with water and carry it with you. Try to have two whole bottles each day. Eat more of the soluble fiber foods like oatmeal and lentil soup because they will help to maintain your blood sugar and minimize your cravings.

During this time be careful about increasing the amount of fruit you are having. As you know, fruits contain sugar and you are trying to decrease your sugar intake. Don't eat more than two pieces a day if you are going to continue eating fruit. Don't have fruit juice during your detox period. Plan what foods you will eat for each of the five days of your detox. You may feel crabby and irritable during this period and may not want to go to the grocery store or have to plan meals. Prepare for this time so you will feel supported and optimistic that you can do it.

As mentioned, your full sugar detox takes about five days. On the first day you'll feel excited about getting started. On day 2 you may begin to feel irritable and edgy. On days 3 and 4 you may be physically uncomfortable with a headache, joint pain or upset stomach. You get these symptoms because you have beta-endorphin receptor sites in other places than your brain. When they don't get the "drug" they are used to, they let you know with symptoms. You may feel irritable, angry, tense or jittery. You may have difficulty concentrating or remembering things. You may wonder why you ever started this detox in the first place.

Day 4, the hardest day, will be crucial. If you get really uncomfortable, have a piece of fruit. No, don't eat four bananas. One will do. Or have an apple or some strawberries. Don't have raisins or figs, even if they call to you. Remember, you are close to being done, so hang in there. If you can manage to get through it, on day 5 you'll feel great! You'll have energy and will feel more stable than you can remember. Coming through a sugar detox will feel good.

Your detox may take a little longer or a little shorter depending on how much you reduce your sugar intake before you start this last phase. Obviously, if you had already taken most things out over time, this phase will be pretty simple. If you decide to be dramatic and go from everything to nothing (which I did myself and *don't* recommend that you do), you will have a dramatic detox—you will feel terrible, then wonderful. At any rate, when you have completed the process, you should feel good.

After you have completed your sugar detox, allow yourself some time to get used to your new way of eating. Keep doing your food journal and let yourself notice how your food plan is going. Stay steady. Keep eating lots of protein, "brown stuff" and "green stuff." Keep eating three meals a day at regular intervals. Keep taking your vitamins. And enjoy how you feel. Alcoholics Anonymous talks about living "one day at a time." With sugar recovery, one day at a time won't work. You will need to live your recovery one choice at a time.

Many people ask me about using "diet" products while they are going off of sugar. Aspartame (Nutrasweet) is made from an amino acid called phenylalanine, and you can have an addictive response to it. Aspartame is used because it tastes sweet. The sweet taste evokes beta-endorphin and we want to reduce beta-endorphin priming by staying away from sweet things.

Notice your own response to diet products. Do you keep a stash of Diet Coke in your refrigerator? Do you look forward to lunch so you can have your diet drink? Do you have a Diet Pepsi on your desk at 9 A.M.? Do you feel relief, satisfaction and physical well-being within ten minutes of having your diet dose? Do you resist the idea of giving it up? If you answer "yes" to any of these questions, you know what this means.

In the first stages after detox, don't think about never having sugar again. That concept is a killer. Don't even try to consider it. Just let yourself stay focused on one choice at a time. Don't even stretch it to one day at a time.

You will have to make food choices every day, many times a day. Going off sugars is a very big deal. Give yourself the recognition and credit for doing a fabulous job which is very difficult. Bravo for you!

Chapter 10

Sticking with It

After you have had a chance to work with your plan for a while, even after you have successfully completed Steps 1 through 6, you may still find that you have a hard time. Three meals a day sounds easy enough, but somehow three meals just don't happen every day. You have good intentions but find it hard to follow through on your program. Let's look at some of the obstacles which may get in the way.

Almost all of the people who start this process are amazed to look at their eating patterns. The usual response is, "I never realized how I was eating." If you notice yourself making lots of excuses about why you don't eat right, listen carefully. The excuses can tell you a whole lot about your inner voices and the "shoulds" you associate with eating. Very gently, without judgment, go back to your food journal and take a look. If you don't eat three meals a day, figure out what factors are preventing following through on your commitment.

Here are some of the patterns that might be developing. Check the ones which apply to you and then read further in the sections which follow.

You may have problems with your eating patterns:
- I can't stand the idea of breakfast.
- I prefer to "graze."
- I don't feel hungry.

You may have time constraints that affect when and how you eat:
- I don't have time.
- I'm too busy.
- My work schedule won't allow it.
- I'm always late in the morning.
- I have to eat out.

You may have financial constraints to consider:
- I don't have a place to prepare food.
- I don't have the money to buy special foods.

You may lack skills related to food:
- I don't know how to cook.
- I eat in front of the TV.

You may have feelings about food that affect your behavior:
- I hate grocery shopping.
- I hate to cook.
- I don't want to eat alone.
- I feel overwhelmed.

Or maybe all of these affect you. Let's go through these patterns one at a time.

Problems with Your Eating Patterns

There can be many reasons you are not able to stick to your food plan. You may not like the idea of breakfast, you may have other habits that conflict with the plan, or you may just be hungry in between meals. Let's look at these:

❑ **I can't stand the idea of breakfast.** Breakfast is a funny meal for people who are sugar sensitive. You, like 95 percent of the clients in the drunk-driving program, may rarely eat breakfast. You may have convinced yourself that it takes too much time, you have to get to work or to school or whatever. You do not feel hungry.

Often you wake up with a headache, feeling a little (or a lot) off, and are not the slightest bit interested in eating until after the coffee and the doughnut (or even the bagel with nonfat cream cheese). You may be in withdrawal first thing in the morning. Your body may have adjusted to a certain level of sugar in the evening. Your brain expects this level. When the sugar level drops, the brain responds with symptoms that make you feel uncomfortable. You may feel irritable and edgy, and have an upset stomach.

Who could eat breakfast feeling like that? But this feeling is the very reason that you need breakfast more than most people.

❑   **I prefer to "graze."** Many people who start this program eat like grazers without realizing it before reading this book. As you work with the food journal, you may see that you tend to eat throughout the day. You may not know why this is. Or you may be "always hungry," or you just can't take time to make a meal, or you don't want to bother.

Often a problem for people who are alcoholic or addicted to sugar, grazing provides no experience with starting and stopping. You just sort of ooze through the day. You have no eating pattern of saying, "Okay, I'm done." Eating three meals a day requires a behavior change that says, "Pay attention to time!" Stop what you are doing and start a meal. Stop when you are finished eating. Starting and stopping is very good training for sugar-sensitive people.

Sometimes people who have low blood sugar (hypoglycemia) hear that they should have six small meals a day instead of three large ones. Six meals a day is not the best solution for someone who has an addictive biochemistry. You need to learn to start and stop eating. If you need to snack between meals, then do so intentionally. It is important that you pay attention to your patterns.

❑   **I don't feel hungry.** For years Suzanne's counselors suggested that she not eat if she wasn't hungry. "Wait until your body signals you," they would say. "The body knows when to eat." But Suzanne never got hungry until at least 1 P.M., so she usually skipped breakfast. After having lunch she wouldn't be hungry again until 9 P.M. It seemed as if her hunger thermostat wasn't working.

But Suzanne stuck with this food plan anyway and ate her three meals a day at regular intervals. After about six months a strange thing happened. She was hungry when she woke up in the morning. She was hungry at noon and before dinner. And if she didn't eat enough, her body told her so with clear signals: hunger pangs. At first she was very distressed by the feeling of hunger. She didn't know what it was. She thought something was wrong with her stomach and called me in a panic. Then she learned what a healthy body does when it is hungry. A healthy body tells you to eat.

But many sugar-sensitive people have their thermostats stuck in the on or off position. If your thermostat is stuck at "on," you might say you are hungry all the time. If your thermostat is stuck at "off," you might say you are never hungry. You, like Suzanne, may not know what being hungry feels like. Hunger is a very specific physiological feeling: your stomach growls and your body seeks food. If you don't have these feelings, you may be feeling something else, such as withdrawal, emotional longing or boredom. Learn to differentiate what real hunger is.

Time Constraints

❏ **I don't have time.** Of course you don't have time. This is why you have gotten into trouble in the first place. You will learn how to *create* time. First, you will just set aside a few minutes three times a day. Maybe 10 minutes of paying attention to your food and consciously eating to start with. Usually, when people start eating real foods their bodies respond very positively. In the beginning, you may be able to find only 10 minutes for your meal, but you will find that you like the experience so much that soon you may be willing to give it 15 minutes, and so on, until you have created a real mealtime.

❏ **I'm too busy.** When you feel you are too busy to pay attention to your food, think about what is really important to you. It may be that you are too busy to make any changes in your life. You may not be willing to let go of anything you are doing in order to make room for paying attention to your food. It is okay to choose this, but be honest with yourself about the choices you are making. Being "too busy" can also reflect an unfocused and scattered mind, which is one of the symptoms of low serotonin. You may find that by taking the time to make changes to your food, you end up being able to get everything done and in significantly less time.

❑ **My work schedule won't allow it.** Many, many people come in and tell me that their work schedule just won't allow them to break away for a meal. You catch something from the deli downstairs or munch on crackers or yogurt at your desk. You grab something from the lunch truck or eat a bite in the car. Mealtime is not a priority for you.

But the first steps in this program demand that you at least consider that eating is important. Try to schedule your meals as if they were time with your most important friend. Taking time for eating is the key to doing this program well. If your company culture doesn't encourage taking time for a meal, change the culture! Get creative on this one. Or if your coworkers eat at their desks and you are not ready to strike a blow for freedom by taking your lunch outside and sitting in the park while you eat, then pack a meal the night before so you can at least eat a healthy meal at your desk.

Making time to eat gives your body the message that it is important. Making sure that your body gets taken care of will reinforce the idea that you are in relationship to it. If you say to your partner or child, "I love you," but you never spend any time with him or her, what message are you really sending? This is what you have been doing with your body. No time means no love.

Create the time for a meal and your body will reward you by feeling healthy, whole and in balance.

❑ **I'm always late in the morning.** Explore what is behind your perennial lateness. Are you super-tired when you get up? Do you not want to go to work? Do you feel like a slug and can't function until you have had some coffee? Once you understand what makes you late, you can decide to take steps to change it. You may choose not to do

Eating on the Run

Rule #1: *Always plan what and when you are going to eat.* Think through your day *before* you leave the house. Plan your danger spots. Take your food. Always keep a plastic bag of your protein powder with you. Put some in your glove compartment or your briefcase. Carry a knife to deal with apples and cheese. Take your power shake in a thermos or take some of last night's dinner as a cold meal in a container.

Of course there may be times when you've forgotten to plan and you find yourself in trouble, in which case go to . . .

Rule #2: *Use your backup plan.* Go into a convenience store, grocery store, deli or even fast-food restaurant. Find something good to eat before the candy bar hops into your mouth. Raisins won't do. Carry this list with you so you know what to get when you are tired, crabby or desperate. Add your own ideas.

- An apple, 2 cheese sticks and a handful of almonds
- A carton of milk with 2 Tbs. of protein powder
- Cottage cheese and an orange
- Sliced turkey, Swiss cheese, avocado and tomato slices
- Chili in a cup and a baked potato
- A baked potato with broccoli and cheese
- A Caesar salad with extra turkey
- Triscuits or whole grain crackers and peanut butter
- A carton of plain yogurt with 10 almonds and $\frac{1}{2}$ cup fresh strawberries
- 2 hard-boiled eggs and an orange
- Shredded wheat and milk in a little box, a banana and a hard-boiled egg
- Breakfast burrito with eggs, beans and cheese. (Use a whole wheat tortilla if you can.)
- A turkey sandwich and a pear
- Chinese food—beef and broccoli and rice. Ask them to hold the MSG and the sugar.
- Ricotta cheese and $\frac{1}{2}$ cup strawberries
- A roast chicken breast with salad
- Spinach salad with tofu chunks
- Egg salad on a whole grain bagel
- Cream cheese, lox on a whole grain bagel
- Chicken taco with lettuce, tomatoes and cheese

anything, but at least you will be deciding rather than simply being a victim of always being late.

❑ **I have to eat out.** Eating out doesn't need to be a problem with this food plan. You can eat at fast-food joints, fancy restaurants or the local deli. After you learn what foods make sense for you and your needs, you can put together meals that fit your plan regardless of where and how you get them.

Eating out is either a disaster that sabotages your plan each time you go out or a real joy and a fun time to share with your friends or family. Plan where to go and identify the options for eating. Keep a number of restaurants that serve foods you can eat up your sleeve, so if your friends suggest going out you can suggest them. But even if you go someplace you have never been, think through what you might have before you go in. Most places serve fish and chicken and will very happily give you additional vegetables if you ask for them.

Plan what you will do if your friends intend to eat dessert. Remember the principle of abundance rather than deprivation. Look at the menu to see what is being served. If fresh fruit is in season, ask the server if you can get some fresh strawberries. At the very worst simply ask for a cup of decaf coffee to enjoy while your friends are having dessert.

Some restaurants have overwhelming cues. One place in my town, for example, is known for its desserts. They practically sing from the lavish dessert case, calling out like sirens to tempt the patrons. If you are feeling at all wobbly don't go into singing restaurants!

Also avoid Thai restaurants; they cook with large amounts of sugar. Chinese restaurants do as well, but may be willing to hold the sugar if asked. You will be surprised at how different many Chinese dishes taste if cooked without sugar. Many people who are sugar sensitive love sushi and tell me how healthy it is. Remember that the rice served with sushi is held together with a sugar binder. No wonder we love it so much! So go to Japanese restaurants, but order fewer California rolls; have less rice and more fish.

Airplane food is harder since there are few choices and it is hard to count on getting sufficient protein. Most airline meals are high in refined carbohydrates and are simply not satisfying for your type of food plan. Order special meals so you will know what you are getting. Take food with you. Plan your favorite things. Get plastic containers and prepare whatever foods or meal will make you feel really nourished. Enjoy your home-cooked meal while your fellow passengers eat prepackaged foods.

Traveling demands the most attention. Always take protein powder with you in a plastic bag. If you get stuck somewhere without being able to get the foods you need, you can always make up a power shake (see recipe on page 114 in Chapter 7).

Financial Constraints

❑ **I don't have a place to prepare food.** You may live somewhere that doesn't have a kitchen. Or you may be on the road all the time. Be creative about how to get the food you want to eat. Yes, you can get fast food which will allow you to do this food plan. You can eat out of your car if you need to. You can eat on the trail or in a boat. Shift your focus from the foods you *can't* get to the foods you *can* and incorporate them into your personalized food plan. We will talk more about this later.

❑ **I don't have the money to buy special foods.** If you don't have a lot of money, going to the grocery store can be uncomfortable because it reminds you that you can't get the things you want. Sometimes when we have uncomfortable or painful feelings we turn to sweet foods to help us feel better. You may be spending money on doughnuts or Cap'n Crunch cereal and not really thinking about it. Buying foods like lentil soup and oatmeal will actually cost less and give you more food value.

Many high-protein foods cost more than foods like pasta, but not all of them do. Eggs are a great buy, and bean and cheese or chicken burritos can provide good protein. Go back to Chapters 8 and 9 to get ideas for foods you can buy or make that are not expensive and will give you the nourishment you need. You will see that you can spend the same amount of money on day-old doughnuts or on a can of chili, but one of them will leave you depressed, impulsive and tired, while the other will make you energetic, optimistic and self-confident. Take your choice!

Lack of Skills

❑ **I don't know how to cook.** Some people get to adulthood and they truly have no idea how to cook.

Learning to cook is easy. The first step is acknowledging that you don't know how. Then do some very specific things.

First, look around you and see who does know how to cook well. Then ask that person to teach you. Tell him you haven't a clue about cooking and you want to start with baby steps. Learn to cook an egg. Learn to boil water, to make oatmeal. Go to a bookstore and ask the staff person to show you the children's cookbooks. Go to the library and ask the librarian for the cookbook section. Choose the book that feels right for you. If you are not comfortable reading, get a book with lots of pictures. If you enjoy reading, choose a book that tells you how to cook the kind of food you really love. Find one cookbook that is about foods you really, really like to eat. Watch cooking programs on TV or get a cooking video that will show you what to do.

Once you've got a cookbook you like, try to follow one recipe and see what happens. Start with something easy enough so you don't get stuck. See if you can master making scrambled eggs or frying a hamburger. Try the same recipe over and over until you get the hang of it. Experiment with one thing—like scrambled eggs—so you can begin to see what variables make a difference in how a food looks or tastes. What happens if you add grated cheese to the eggs? Or cream cheese? Or curry powder?

Begin to notice what you like: what tastes, what texture, what colors, what smells. Most sugar-sensitive people have never noticed these things. In the past, you were primarily interested in getting foods which satisfied your sugar cravings or stopped your feelings of withdrawal.

When you first start to cook, some of the food you make will be just horrible. That's normal! The first time I made fried chicken, I didn't know that the chicken had to cook on the inside as well as being brown on the outside. I proudly served it to my new husband, thinking I was very cool. The chicken had the indecency to bleed all over the plate. It was pretty horrible. But now I know how to cook chicken just fine.

Every new thing you do begins with learning how. People who love to cook will be delighted to show you what to do. But you have to ask them.

❑   **I eat in front of the TV.** Eating in front of the TV is better than not eating at all. However, eating in front of the TV does not lend itself to forming a relationship to your food. How can you connect with what you are eating or how you are eating or how it tastes if you're thinking about what is playing on the tube?

Much of television is very fast-paced. It activates adrenaline. When you're eating while watching an exciting show, you don't have to notice how you feel. You can leave your cares and attention behind. You may be inhaling your food without thinking about it at all. You may be eating a huge amount and not even notice. You may not like what you are eating.

Ideally, you can learn to know what is on your plate, how you feel about every single food on it. Sit down at a table and eat a meal. Look at the food, taste it, feel the texture, think about where it came from, who planted it, where it grew, how it got to you. Think about how it was cooked. Do you like eating this food? When you have found your stride, you will notice and enjoy every meal you eat.

Feelings About Food

Feelings have a huge impact on your eating patterns. Some of these feelings may be connected to old stories or images from your childhood. Eating may even have a negative emotional context for you. It may be helpful for you to explore these things with a counselor who is supportive, kind and patient and who can help you sort out the many layers of what you feel. As your body chemistry gets stable from doing the food plan, you may find that it is far easier to know which are the true emotional blocks that need to be healed and which were just the negative feelings that came from eating sugars and refined carbohydrates.

However, at this point, it is important to honor some of the feelings that are related to doing the food plan. Let's take a look at these:

❑ **I hate grocery shopping.** Some people absolutely hate going into grocery stores. Like many of the feelings you examined in earlier steps, get to know what is behind this avoidance. Think about what part of shopping you hate. Is it thinking about what you need, making a list, having to choose, not having money? Sort out which part of shopping you hate. Then do some problem-solving on that specific part.

If making lists aggravates you, try drawing pictures. Or you can make a map of the store. Or you can simply think breakfast, lunch, dinner and remember what to buy that way. Be creative. If you hate having to choose different foods, get the same foods every time you go. You don't need to be a gourmet cook. It's your food. Do what makes sense for you.

If you hate standing in line or even going into the grocery store, you can find ways to deal with this. If you have a computer, a number of shopping services allow you to order on-line and have your groceries delivered right to you. Or you can hire a high school student to go shopping for you. Or trade with a friend: you do the laundry or watch the kids while he does your grocery shopping. You will still have to plan what to get, but you won't have to go into that store.

❑ **I hate to cook.** Some people truly hate to cook. They hate making a mess or they feel stupid because what they make tastes terrible. Or they simply think cooking is dumb. There is nothing in this food plan that says you have to cook. Just acknowledge that you hate to cook and move on from there.

If you don't want to cook, you need to find other ways to get the foods you need at the times you need them. Here are some alternatives for you:

• You could hire a cook.
• You could find a boyfriend or girlfriend who is a fabulous cook.

- You can find a great takeout place.
- You can check out the local deli.
- You can learn to make great choices at fast-food places.
- You can learn what nutritious foods at the supermarket require no cooking (some might require boiling water).
- You can eat foods that don't have to be cooked.
- You can use frozen or canned foods that are easy to heat and eat.
- You can cook a huge amount once a week and eat the leftovers each day or make two or three dishes on your cooking day for more variety.
- You can ask your parents to send you food in a basket (make sure they know what you are eating so you don't get your mother's favorite chocolate cake).
- You can figure out four basic meals that you can stand to make and simply rotate through them.

❑ **I don't want to eat alone.** Sometimes people eat in front of the TV because they live alone and hate the idea of eating by themselves. Honor this feeling. Instead of using the TV for company, however, pretend you are making a meal for someone you love. Then sit and enjoy it with your imaginary buddy. Imagine she feels really blessed by your taking time to shop for the food, prepare it with care and spend the time with her over dinner.

Imagine now that this friend is actually a special part of you. She hasn't had any time with you for years. She has been left behind or she has had to sit in the other room while you watch TV and eat. Think of how joyful she is going to feel if you begin to spend time with her.

❑ **I feel overwhelmed.** Very often feeling overwhelmed is a result of how you have been eating. As we've seen, feeling overwhelmed can have a clear biochemical basis. As you change your food, life will feel more manageable. As you get more stable and focused, you may wonder why the task that felt so overwhelming seemed hard at all. But while this peace of mind may come in time, right now you still feel overwhelmed.

When you feel overwhelmed, you tune out and you don't deal with problems. Then they just get worse. So start with the very first step—writing in your food journal. This will help you see what contributes to feeling overwhelmed. Not eating or eating lots of sugar are both killers in the "overwhelmed" world. But you won't see that for yourself until you have a record of your food and your feelings. Write diligently for a week, even if it seems like a huge task. Then put on your detective hat and start figuring out what's going on with your food plan and with your life.

All of the Above

If you feel like "All of the Above" are obstacles, you sound like a person who has a problem with sugar or alcohol. Keep working on your food plan and you'll be okay. Make a list of the things that contribute to your not being able to eat three times a day. Start a dialogue with yourself. See if there are solutions you can find for each of the things that are obstacles for you. While you are working on these obstacles, keep your food journal (Step 1), eat three meals a day at regular intervals (Step 2), take your vitamins (Step 3) and make a commitment to eating the recommended protein at each meal (Step 4).

After you have got these four steps under your belt, you will experience a significant change in the way you feel. Eating regularly keeps your blood sugar level constant. An even blood sugar level will have a huge impact on how you feel throughout the day. You will be energetic instead of tired, focused instead of confused and easygoing instead of irritable.

Dealing with Special Situations

As you become more and more skilled in doing your food plan, you will become more adept at dealing with special situations that come up. But in the beginning it will be easier for you to master the plan if you are a little more rigid about it. Here are some suggestions to keep you on track:

Keep temptation to a minimum around sweets. Remember the power of priming, which we discussed in Chapter 5. One cookie or one taste of chocolate pudding won't throw you totally off your plan. But it will prime your brain to want more. Having something sweet "just this once" will activate an endorphin response and set off craving for more sweets. If you are not paying attention, this craving will catch you off guard and you will soon be sliding into relapse.

Be forewarned and be prepared to protect yourself and your recovery. There will be times when you will have to make an informed choice about whether to maintain your food plan or not. Preparation is your best defense. We'll talk about how to handle specific situations in this section, but the main thing you'll need to do is think ahead, identify all the possibilities and always have a backup plan.

Traveling

Keeping on a food plan when you travel is hard. Think through the staples that you can always get on the road. Eggs, tuna fish, chicken, beef, cottage cheese, nuts, potatoes, salad. Have a few basic foods that you can always find, even if you are on the thruway in Indiana.

Don't leave it to chance. If you know or even suspect that the only options will be fast foods that don't include protein or any complex carbohydrates, pack your food and take it with you. Get a cooler, keep a stash of food in your car or hotel room. Bring protein powder and apples and cheese. Know where you are going and what the options will be.

Traveling in a foreign country can be even more problematic. Many cultures are in love with foods that are not the best for you. Teatime in England is seductive. Pasta in Italy will sound wonderful. French bread will call you. Put on your adventure hat and *plan* what choices you have before you are hungry and tired. Ask the local chefs to prepare something that works for you. You can have cheese and crackers instead of tea cakes, grilled vegetable vinaigrette instead of pasta. There isn't really an alternative for French bread. We all know this. If I pretended there was, I would lose my credibility with you. I, like you, know there is no substitute. You will just have to hold your impulse and smile.

Parties

Find out what food will be served at a party before you go. Will there be nonalcoholic drinks? Will there be sugar-free drinks? Will there be any foods not loaded with sugars?

If there won't be food that is appropriate for you, take something with you. Always, always be prepared. If you are going to a potluck, bring a dish that you know you can eat. Make sure to get yourself a helping of it before everyone else discovers your special dish. You

---

Going to Aunt Sue's House for Potluck

Plan: Take your own chicken and broccoli casserole.

Reality: You forget the casserole.

Backup Plan: Choose food to give you enough protein. Eat vegetables and salad.

Reality: She serves homemade pasta, warm garlic bread, salad and a fabulous dessert. She is thrilled that you are there to enjoy her cooking.

Disaster Plan: Smile. Eat some pasta and lots of salad. Don't tell yourself that since you are having it, you might as well go whole hog and eat everything. Forgo the bread and pass on the dessert. Tell your aunt that you aren't doing desserts these days. Have two slices of turkey when you go home and *pay attention* the next day. You will want muffins for breakfast, bagels for a snack, warm bread for lunch, cookies in the afternoon, wine for dinner and dessert afterwards. Just go back to your plan.

---

could be left with your dish cleaned out and have no other healthy options to eat!

Make sure you get your meal (and your protein) no matter what. Plan for this. If you are going to a dinner party, ask the hostess what will be served before you go. You can always choose to eat what fits into your food plan without making a big deal of it. But if the menu is pasta and salad with a wonderful dessert, you will be in trouble. Salad is not enough of a meal. Always think ahead. Eat something before leaving home if you have to. Do not leave yourself in the lurch. Have a plan, a backup plan and a disaster plan.

Holidays

Holidays, oh, holidays. Soon you will discover that sugar, white flour and alcohol are the center of American holiday celebrations. Birthdays, Thanksgiving, Christmas, New Year's, Hanukkah, Halloween. Food galore!

Healthy holidays for people who are sugar sensitive take careful planning and require loving support. If you don't think holidays through ahead of time, you will either slip off your food plan or feel a huge sense of frustration, regret and remorse when you are left out of traditions that have meant a lot to you.

Prepare for the first holiday after designing your food plan very carefully. Practice the expected rituals. If birthday cakes are a big part of your family tradition, plan a way to get a sugar-free cake with whole grains. Yes, there are options for this, but you have to do some homework and some choosing. Look in the library for whole grain or sugar-free cookbooks. Make sure to notice what "sugar-free" means. Some cookbooks offer sugar-free recipes made with huge amounts of dried fruits.

In the same way, some of the choices billed as "sugar-free" in grocery stores actually have huge amounts of fruit sugars. This won't work for you, but foods like unsweetened applesauce or juice-sweetened carrot cake may be just fine and not trigger you at all. As in other special situations, know ahead of time what you are going to eat. Try out the recipe first so you don't end up with your crowning glory tasting like a piece of cardboard, and making your family mad at you because the holiday isn't the same and you are to blame for the change.

If someone else plans the holiday feast, decide before the event what you will eat. Make sure you don't go to the party hungry. Smells and sights will trigger you. Practice the situation before it happens. Know your plan.

Halloween will remind you of pillowcases filled with candy. You will remember lying in bed with a flashlight sorting your treasures. Halloween can be redeemed but it is hard. Put the emphasis on the ritual rather than the candy. Have your children help with choices. Have them go trick or treating for UNICEF and hold a party with such activities as bobbing for apples and playing other games. Hold your ground about boundaries and don't buy candy for all the neighborhood children and then eat it yourself.

Thanksgiving is tough. So much of the love of Thanksgiving comes with dessert. Think about whether you can make a dessert that will work for you. Get creative. Brainstorm with your family about nonsugar options. Enlisting their support will make the process a celebration of sharing rather than a source of either resentment or denial.

Christmas and Hanukkah can be difficult as well. Cookies, special breads and candy are central to how these times are celebrated. You will need to reframe the holiday to fit your plan. You can do it by developing new holiday rituals that don't revolve around food. Hot chocolate can be made without sugar (use baking cocoa and saccharine), and hot cider with cinnamon is a delicious alternative to mulled wine.

Sometimes sugar-sensitive people decide that they will just "blow off" the day and eat what they want. You may choose to do this, but prepare yourself for what will happen. If you have been careful about what you are eating and have cut way down on sugars, remember that you will be in a highly upregulated state. Your brain will have opened up more serotonin and beta-endorphin receptors to compensate for your reduction in sugar use from having been on your food plan.

Those receptors are just sitting there waiting for a sugar hit. When you eat a lot of sugar—ice cream and cake, a dozen Christmas cookies, Aunt Sharon's noodle kugel—the beta-endorphin receptors are going to go wild. You will feel incredible. Life will be wonderful, fine, warm and mellow. You will feel beta-endorphin euphoria and serotonin satisfaction. It will be wonderful. For a few hours.

The next day you will feel terrible. All those receptors will be screaming because they are now empty and want more. What's more, your serotonin level will have dropped again and you'll be low on impulse control. Here's the dilemma. Just as you are in the midst of this heightened receptor activation and craving, there will still be lots of good stuff around to eat. You may also experience a big sugar hangover. You may feel as if you had been drinking all night even though you didn't drink anything. Your cells will be telling you that relief is only a bite away.

The leftovers will call to you big time. A turkey sandwich on white bread, stuffing, a piece of apple pie. Your brain will try to convince you that "just one more" won't hurt anything. After all, yesterday made you feel good and nothing awful happened. Remember there are no negative consequences right away. They come later after you have lost the month and feel terrible. If you have been on the food plan and then relapse, you will feel far worse than before you started the plan.

Remember that your brain chemistry is totally different now. You don't have the same latitude to muck around that you once did. Your brain is in an upregulated state because you are eating less sugar now. Over time, this will change as your brain gets balanced and your lifestyle evokes slow, regular beta-endorphin release through such activities as meditation and exercise. But early on, when you relapse, your craving will be greater, your withdrawal more severe. Your emotional state will be far more vulnerable because you know how it feels to be free of sugar. You will be angry at yourself. Your "sugar feelings" —confusion, anger, restlessness and fatigue—will seem enormous and feel very real. You won't be able to talk to other people about what is going on because you will either feel guilty or disconnected to others (thanks to your now low beta-endorphin level). Your friends who still drink or eat lots of sugar may even encourage your relapse because you are back to what they feel is normal.

Facing the Challenges

Remember to be gentle with yourself through these challenging times. I have been working on my food recovery for many years and I still find holidays difficult. Those little Christmas cookies with the green icing still call my name. I still struggle with wanting pecan pie at Thanksgiving. Know that all of us who are sugar sensitive—*all of us*—go through this process.

Healing your sugar sensitivity is not like abstaining from alcohol and drugs. You do not and cannot put food away forever. You must make choices about what you will eat several times a day. You may be faced with a hundred choices in just one day. This is really hard no matter how you look at it. And if you are in a vulnerable, upregulated state, it will be even harder. This is why having support is critical. Line up your ducks before you are faced with these situations. Enlist the aid of your friends and supporters.

Remember to have a plan, a backup plan and a disaster plan. If you get into trouble and you didn't have a plan, stop and make one. Go back to your food journal. Write everything down—your food, your physical sensations and your feelings. Do one meal at a time. You will be okay. Things will settle down. I have never met anyone who had achieved a week of being totally clean who didn't *always* go back to her journal. All your molecules will remember recovery. They will remind you and draw you back. No matter how far you stray along the way, the power of recovery will call you home.

Trust your body. Once you know the story underneath what is happening, your molecules will yearn for balance, care and healing. Along with the cravings for sugar will come a longing for wholeness. This longing is the real power of the work we are doing. I have seen the transformation over and over and over. Nonpunitive, loving and very, very supportive, this program will carry you through good times and hard times. Go back to basics when you need to and work the plan. You'll make it!

And remember, if you slip it is not a big deal. This is a lifelong process. You do not have a "sobriety" date to mark that you will never eat sugars again. This is a process. You move more and more in relationship to your body. Each slip and each return to the plan reinforces your commitment to pay attention and find a solution that works for you over the long haul. This plan will ask you to reframe all the negative messages you have carried for many, many years. The day you started your food journal marked a shift in your relationship to your body. Trust your intention.

Chapter 11

✦

So You Drink Coffee, Smoke and Stay Fat?

As you have gained skill with your food plan, become more biochemically stable and started to feel better, you may find that you are ready to tackle some of the other addictions in your life. Start by once again being tender. You don't need to attach any negative judgments to having addictions. It's not your fault. This is about biochemistry leading you into behaviors. As you understand more and more what is going on, you will be able to work with your biochemistry and change your behavior. Use the same process that has been working so well. Use your journal. Take it slowly and maintain a sense of humor.

Caffeine

You may not even think of caffeine as a drug, but let's take a look at how it affects your body. Caffeine creates temporary alertness and clarity. It increases your heart rate and gastric secretions. By decreasing the blood flow to your brain, caffeine also helps to relieve headaches. It has prompt and powerful diuretic effects, causing you to lose stored water. When you feel bloated, caffeine helps you return to normal. Caffeine also helps your bowels to move. Many people depend upon that morning cup of coffee to get them "moving" in more ways than one.

Remember these physical effects. They will all change as you go off caffeine. As always, you will want to continue to make connections between what goes into your body and how you feel emotionally.

How Caffeine Affects You

Caffeine is a powerful drug. The amount of caffeine found in the brain is directly related to the amount of caffeine taken. The peak level occurs 30 to 45 minutes after taking it and then about 15 percent is excreted each hour. This means it takes a full six hours for all the drug to leave your body. Caffeine affects a number of neurochemicals in your brain. One of these, adenosine, is responsible for quieting you down. Caffeine is shaped like adenosine and can sit in the adenosine receptor site. This blocks the adenosine message. The net effect is that you feel more alert. Caffeine also stimulates the release of two other brain chemicals that make you feel really good, norepinephrine and dopamine. Norepinephrine is a kind of adrenaline. By activating this chemical, caffeine gives you a hit of energy and gets you mobilized. When dopamine is released the parts of the brain called the reward centers are activated and you feel really good. Amphetamines and cocaine also have a dopamine effect in these same reward centers. Caffeine is a drug which affects these same places.

Since caffeine is a drug, you develop tolerance to it. You need more of it to continue feeling good over time, and you don't feel good if you don't have it. The need to feel better can move you from a relatively moderate and comfortable use of caffeine to a serious addiction. Like other drugs, caffeine can create a powerful physical dependence. Notice how much better you feel after that first cup of coffee in the morning. After you come to depend on caffeine, you no longer feel high when you use it. You simply look for relief from your withdrawal symptoms.

As a socially accepted drug, caffeine remains a large part of cultural socialization. The impact of caffeine is growing. Not too long ago a new coffee store opened in my community. The first week the hours were 7 A.M. to 10 P.M. Three weeks later the hours were 6 A.M. to 11

P.M. Now the store is open from 5 A.M. to midnight. Eleven thousand cups of coffee beverages are served at this store *in a week*. Every few months a new promotion comes out—a bigger size, a frosted mocha, extra shots. At most coffee bars a whole language has arisen around the process of serving the coffee. "Double, low-fat, iced macchiato to go. Triple regular latte for here." New flavors, new textures, a whole culture around caffeine has sprung up.

The patterns are the same as with sugar. You feel wonderful. For a while. Then all of a sudden 3 P.M. is unbearable. You have to have a cup of coffee. You start leaving the pot on, you buy an espresso machine. You have one at work. This kind of behavior is about addiction and relief from withdrawal. When your brain isn't getting the drug it has adapted to, you don't feel well.

You probably don't make the connection between your caffeine intake and your irritability. You haven't noticed the relationship between the timing of your withdrawal symptoms and your inability to focus and think clearly. What you do remember is the times you have felt good. And you will do anything to try to maintain those feelings.

Your Caffeine Use

The first step in dealing with your caffeine use is to notice how much and when you use it. Assess the amount of caffeine you are using each day and each week. Take out your food journal and read it with an eye to caffeine. Start by highlighting the foods and drinks that contain caffeine. Make a separate list of each of these.

The chart on page 170 identifies the major sources of caffeine in the average diet.

After you have highlighted all the caffeine you consume in a day, calculate the total milligrams of caffeine you are getting. Make sure to adjust the fluid ounces of your drink to the 12-ounce portion just noted. If you have three Cokes in 32-ounce containers in a day, you are having 96 ounces of Coke. Since one ounce of Coke has about 4 mg of caffeine, you are having almost 400 mg of caffeine. If you have 4 grande (16-ounce) cups of coffee in a day, you are having around

1100 mg of caffeine. Were you surprised to see the actual amount of caffeine you use? Had you realized all the sources of caffeine in your daily diet?

The effect of your caffeine dosage will depend upon your body weight. High caffeine use can induce symptoms of anxiety—a racing heartbeat, shakiness, diarrhea, stomach pain, spots in front of the eyes, ringing in the ears or a tingling in your fingers or toes. All too often when people seek treatment for symptoms like these, no one ever asks how much caffeine they use. High intakes of caffeine can produce symptoms that are indistinguishable from those of anxiety

Source	Amount	Caffeine (mg)
coffee, brewed	12 oz.	206
coffee, instant	12 oz.	114
coffee, espresso (one shot)	1 oz.	71
coffee, double latte (two shots)	2 oz.	142
coffee, brewed decaf	12 oz.	4
coffee, instant decaf	12 oz.	3
tea, brewed	12 oz.	71
tea, iced lemon flavor	12 oz.	39
cocoa	12 oz.	11
Mountain Dew	12 oz.	55
Diet Coke	12 oz.	50
Coca-Cola Classic	12 oz.	45
Pepsi	12 oz.	37
Dr Pepper	12 oz.	37
Bromo-Seltzer	1 dose	33
Midol	1 dose	32
Dexatrim	1 dose	200
NoDoz	1 dose	100

esha Food Processor

neurosis. Doctors have been known to prescribe anti-anxiety medication while the patient is still drinking a pot of coffee a day.

If you drink more than three cups of coffee a day, or have more than two shots of espresso or drink more than three glasses of iced tea or have more than three cans of soda with caffeine, proceed more slowly with this next phase of your recovery. Do not quit caffeine cold turkey. Withdrawal from caffeine may bring on headaches, nausea, lethargy, fatigue, difficulty concentrating, lack of energy, inability to work effectively, less sociability, shakiness or irritability. Sometimes people drink a lot of coffee at work and very little on the weekend. Over the weekend they feel terrible and incorrectly attribute these feelings to family problems.

Withdrawal from caffeine is not limited to high users. Some people can be drinking one or two cups of coffee a day and experience caffeine withdrawal. Or they may be drinking a six-pack of Diet Coke, knowing they are cutting out the sugar, but never thinking about the caffeine. Before you start a caffeine detox, use your food journal to help you investigate your use pattern. Remember that when we are dragging around, feeling sleepy, lethargic, disoriented and foggy, a cup of coffee seems like a wonder drug. The problem is that we are using the wonder drug rather than dealing with our need for rest. Resting when we are tired may seem like an outrageous idea. But learning to take care of your body continues to be the focus of the path to recovery.

The other dilemma tied to your caffeine use is the connection to our socialization. Caffeine, especially coffee, is a huge part of the way we connect to others. If you aren't going out for a drink, of course you will go out for coffee. We usually don't invite people out for water. Coffee bars are the wave of new glamour, the good alternative to bars. You may not want to give up coffee because you feel so attached to all these wonderful cues associated with it—the aroma, the taste, and on and on. But remember, you can find ways to have the social and emotional enjoyment connected to the ritual without using the drug. You can go for coffee and have decaf. This maintains the social ritual but keeps you out of trouble. But pay attention to whether the cues are stimulating you to want the real thing. You may need to wait until your neurochemistry quiets down some. You will know the right thing to do.

Going Out for "Coffee"

You can still enjoy the social part of going out. Get the same cup and fill it with something new. Enjoy the ritual part and take out the part that is difficult for you. Let someone else order for you so you don't have to stand by the goodies case. Choose wisely. Ask your body if these will work for you.

- Decaf latte and a whole wheat scone
- Herbal tea (either hot or cold)
- Iced decaf coffee with a little cream
- A little orange juice (3 oz.) in a large glass of sparkling water
- Lemon and water (either hot or cold)

TIP: Focus on the *company* you are with rather than the food.

Go back to your journal and use your awareness skills to identify whether your caffeine use is a problem. If you decide to eliminate caffeine, you can do so with little physical discomfort. Withdrawal symptoms can be avoided by eliminating caffeine gradually.

Eliminating Caffeine

Start with knowing how much caffeine you use and when you use it. Be very clear about identifying your patterns of caffeine use. Now make a plan to cover a month. The first week you are going to decrease the amount of caffeine you use by one-fourth. You can do this by cutting out one-fourth of the number of cups you drink or by substituting decaf for one-fourth of your intake.

If you substitute you have two choices. You could have a decaf drink in place of one-fourth of your regular cups of coffee. That's the hard way. And you probably won't like it because your body will notice that it didn't get any caffeine and will start screaming an hour later. When you have your next cup of the real stuff, you will inhale it in desperation.

A better plan is to substitute one-fourth decaf in each cup you are drinking. Yes, the person at the counter of the coffee store will do this for you. Just ask. Or when you make a pot of coffee for yourself, include one-quarter decaf in the grounds. Now don't cheat and get stronger coffee. Use the same coffee, the same rituals and drink your cup at the same times of the day. If you do it this way, you will hardly notice a change. Remember that your food plan will be supporting your brain chemistry. As you have worked to increase your serotonin level, you will have more impulse control.

The second week, you will do the same thing, only decrease the amount of caffeine by one-half. That means ordering or making every cup of coffee you have half decaf and half regular coffee. Trust me, your body will adjust. Remember abundance rather than deprivation. We are working to get you off caffeine, not take away all that is associated with the emotional and social comfort of going for coffee. You can be creative about this.

The third week, guess what you are going to do? Three-quarters decaf. And the fourth week you will go off caffeine and drink only decaf. Do this for another week. Then decide whether you want to cut down on the decaf. Some women find that they have a negative response to even decaffeinated coffee. If you have cystic breast disease, you may need to cut it out entirely. You may find that it really isn't as important to be having coffee all day. The decaf doesn't have the same charge, does it? It's the drug caffeine that you love.

Your caffeine use may be coming from diet soda. You won't be able to mix decaf with regular as with coffee. Develop a plan for how many sodas you will have in a day. Replace some with caffeine-free drinks. If you can't get the right kind of caffeine-free diet soda from a vending machine, try a different brand. As you go through this process, be attentive to how many "diet" products you are using. Remember that phenylalanine can act like a stimulant in your body. You may be physically addicted to the "diet" chemicals without realizing it. Use your well-developed skills to sort out where the draw is.

Usually when people go off caffeine they don't feel well for a while and then they feel enormously better. The effort was well worth it.

However, going off caffeine may have some problematic effects. If you're depressed, you may be using caffeine to cover your symptoms. When you complete your caffeine detox, you may find it is extremely difficult to get out of bed, that you are tired all the time, you have no energy and you just want to sleep all day. If the food changes have not helped the symptoms either, then it is important for you to seek professional support. You do not have to not feel good.

As you finish your caffeine detox, you may experience some other changes. If you have panic attacks, you may find they improve significantly when you stop using caffeine. If you have anxiety, you may find this is the first symptom which improves. If you suffer from attention deficit disorder (ADD), you may have been using a high caffeine dose to quiet your brain. At high dosage caffeine can create a Ritalin-like effect by overloading the dopamine system and causing the receptors to downregulate. When you stop using caffeine the system upregulates and you may feel less focused and more scattered. However, many people find that the dietary changes they make prior to removing the caffeine significantly affect their mental functioning in a positive way. If you do have ADD, some caffeine may help you in a positive way. Once again, your task is to make sense of what works for you. Using caffeine for the medicinal effects of the drug is very different from using caffeine addictively. Slowing ADD will feel different from dealing with withdrawal. Pay attention.

Also pay attention to what you use with your coffee. You may be drinking coffee for the sugar you add to it. You may be ordering latte for the milk rather than the coffee. After the infamous coffee store opened down the street from me, I found myself planning a daily trip for a latte. Once a day grew to several times. A single "short" developed into a double "grande." I even knew which airports had a branch of this coffee store. I knew the hours, I knew which *barristas* (the gussied-up name for the staff who made the coffee) made the best drink. I knew the location of every store within a hundred-mile radius of my house. This was addiction at its worst.

But it wasn't only the caffeine I was addicted to. I experimented to see if I had the same longing when I drank espresso without the milk. Nope, that little cup of black liquid didn't hold quite the same charge as the warm milk. Another connection to my early story of going to Dairy Queen. Milk and mother. Love. Opioids. Once I saw what was driving my behavior, I decided love can come from better places than a coffee store.

So, eliminate the caffeine first, then take a look at what else is connected to your coffee-drinking habit. Look at what other "drugs," like sugar or milk or croissants or cigarettes, are connected to it. Look at what's important in the ritual of coffee drinking. Look at how much coffee is a part of our social culture. Watch with the same attention that you have used to explore your other issues. If you can retain a sense of humor, you will fare better. This is hard work. Be patient, be tender.

If you notice that smoking is a regular part of your coffee ritual, don't be surprised at the power of the link. Often coffee and cigarettes are so powerfully associated that one will feel incomplete without the other. Unravel the connection and work on eliminating one thing at a time. Start with the caffeine and then work on the nicotine.

Nicotine

Dealing with smoking is a very difficult process. In some ways, nicotine addiction is the most complex of the physical dependencies to deal with. Nicotine affects a greater number of biochemical pathways than most other drugs. It also provides a large number of benefits which seem very persuasive. Quitting smoking will demand knowing the issues involved, coming up with a plan which works and getting the huge amount of support you will need to follow through. If you do smoke now, you already know nicotine's power. No doubt, you have tried to stop many times. You may find that adding in the nutritional piece can provide a support to help you through the most difficult part. Because smoking has become less socially acceptable in many parts of the country, you may find that you have become increasingly isolated in your dependence upon cigarettes. Remember, dealing with any addiction requires having support. It is crucial for you to seek out other people who understand what you are going through and will support your commitment to make a change. People who have never smoked may cheer for your decision to quit, but ex-smokers will be able to truly understand what you are feeling.

How Nicotine Affects You

Nicotine affects a whole cascade of neurochemical responses which include the brain chemicals—dopamine, serotonin, beta-endorphin and norepinephrine. Nicotine makes you high, relieves depression, creates euphoria, suppresses your appetite, increases your metabolism, relaxes you, enhances learning, creates mental focus and increases your ability to solve problems. It sure sounds wonderful, doesn't it? The act of smoking gives you fingertip control over the level and timing of your dosage. How much you smoke, how deeply you inhale and for how long all affect the impact of the nicotine in your brain. Whenever a drug gives you control over these effects, the drug becomes very addictive.

But those seemingly wonderful effects come at a huge price. Smoking kills 400,000 people a year, or more than 1000 people a day! But it is hard to see the consequences of smoking on a daily basis. The impact of smoking on your body is more subtle in the beginning. Addictive use of crack can ruin your life in six months and addictive use of cocaine may do it in three years. Alcohol takes years to wear you down. The negative impact of smoking creeps up on you over a long period of time. You may smell bad, have an ongoing cough, but it doesn't really seem to have an effect except to make you feel better when you do smoke. Then, BAM, you are diagnosed with lung cancer. Even then, your brain may tell you that you need a cigarette to help you cope with the feelings.

Withdrawal from nicotine produces very uncomfortable side effects. The list that follows will tell you all of the uncomfortable symptoms which may emerge with withdrawal. Essentially when you're smoking you feel "good"—that is, focused, clear and relaxed—and when you don't smoke you gain weight, are muddleheaded and feel as if a truck ran over you. You may rationally know it is not good for you, but you are compelled to respond to the intensity of the distress you feel when you are in withdrawal. You want to stop but your body will do anything to get rid of the awful feelings. People who tell you to just stop have no idea of the intensity of these feelings.

Your first step will be to know the power of the drug you are dealing with. You will need to become aware of the physical symptoms

Symptoms of Nicotine Withdrawal

Irritability/frustration/anger	Tightness in chest
Anxiety	Bodily aches and pains
Depression	Tingling sensation in limbs
Hostility	Stomach distress
Impatience	Hunger
Drowsiness	Craving
Fatigue	Performance deficits
Restlessness	Sleep disturbance
Difficulty concentrating	Constipation
Decreased alertness	Sweating
Lightheadedness	Mouth ulcers
Headaches	Increased coughing

which may emerge when you start to withdraw. You need to watch how you use nicotine to handle your feelings, suppress your appetite and enhance your performance. Your recovery plan will need to address each one of these benefits and offer another alternative which works. To quit smoking successfully, you will need to turn up your awareness to a very powerful level. You will need all the detective skills you have.

Use your food journal to get started with this process. Focus on your smoking patterns with the kind of attention you did to look at your sugar use. When and why do you reach for a cigarette? You may feel that your patterns are simply "habit," but when you start to pay attention you will see the power of the negative feelings of withdrawal and the emotional impact of getting relief. Get to know your smoking rhythms and triggers really, really well. Tease out all the reasons you smoke. Notice what increases your craving and what relieves it. Notice the times and places you associate with smoking. Watch for your reflexive reactions. You may always reach for a cigarette under stress. Rosemary stopped smoking twelve years ago. Recently, a car clipped her ankle as she was crossing the road. After the first flurry of activity to make sure she was all right, she sat down. She realized that she really wanted a cigarette. Twelve years later it was still a powerful link to resolving stress.

Learn the difference between your physical and your emotional needs. You have the skills to do this now. These skills have been well practiced for a number of months. Finally, you have a process to help you sort out a plan which can work for you.

Planning a Nicotine Detox

The first step of your detox plan is to separate the physical and emotional components of your nicotine use. I generally recommend that people stop smoking before they go off the drug nicotine. If you give up cigarettes but continue with a nicotine patch or gum, you can deal with the behavior changes you must make without having to deal with the physical withdrawal from nicotine. Explore options. The patch can provide a steady flow of nicotine but the gum allows you to have more control over the rate and flow of the drug in your system. Depending upon your typical cigarette use patterns, you should choose the option which will work best. If you have been smoking at irregular intervals, such as only in the car or only in the evening after work, you may find that the gum works better because your body is used to having the drug at these intervals. If you are used to smoking throughout the day, the patch may work better for you.

However, if you have not done your homework to understand the emotional factors contributing to your nicotine use, the patch may not work. When you are under stress, you will reach for a cigarette to calm you, even if you are using the patch. People who do not smoke cannot understand how someone on the patch can pick up a cigarette. Smokers know better. Everything may feel settled until you hit emotional stress and then you will seek the old comfort of the nicotine. A cigarette will kick up the nicotine level above the resting state created by the patch and you will feel the high that comes with increasing the dose.

This time, however, you can know what is happening. You can choose what you want. You will have increased your serotonin levels so that saying no will be easier. You will have increased your beta-endorphin levels so that you have more confidence and feel less emotionally vulnerable, and therefore less in need of nicotine support. And you have learned to get support in the process. Find other people who have successfully stopped smoking. Talk to them. Reinforce your commitment by being around others who have succeeded.

Plan a detox which fits your style. You may go to a stop smoking clinic at your hospital, you may attend a special workshop, you may attend a behavioral modification class to learn to count and time your cigarettes, you may get hypnotized, or you may simply follow the detox schedule outlined on the box of patches. In fact, you may have already tried any or all of these options. You may be skeptical that it could work this time. Remember, though, that you are bringing both a new awareness and a new brain to the process. The schemes which did not work before may be ideal this time around. Your awareness is entirely different and you have a whole set of new nutritional skills at your disposal.

The specific nutritional supports which will help your detox include increasing your protein levels at each meal (up to .5 gram per pound of body weight) and having some sort of slow carbohydrate every night before you go to bed (to maximize your serotonin). Choose slow carbs so you won't activate your beta-endorphin receptors and prime your interest in smoking. A baked potato with the skin is ideal because it is both a comfort food and a slow carbohydrate. Potato chips or French fries don't count unless they have the skin. Drink lots and lots and lots of water. Increase your vitamin C level to bowel tolerance (to enhance clearing out the garbage put off by the detox), and increase your zinc intake for about a month.

Don't start turning to sugar to ease your discomfort. You may be uncomfortable for several weeks. Go slowly enough so you feel you are in charge. You can either taper or go cold turkey. Just as you did with your sugar detox, pay attention to the style that works for you.

Use your journal to identify the feelings being triggered. Be tender with yourself and know that this detox, like all the others you have done, is a process which will continue over time. The nicest thing about quitting smoking is you will feel so much better. Your lungs will clear, your brain will clear, you will stop coughing, your clothes and house will smell better, your car will stay clean. Things you never noticed will pop up as benefits. Best of all, there are huge health benefits from quitting. Bravo for you!

Losing Weight

Let's turn now to the issue that many of you may struggle with. I know you have been chomping at the bit. You think that being thin is the most important part of the plan. You may be surprised to find this section at the end of the book rather than at the beginning. I am adamant that weight loss must come out of recovery rather than start it. If you have gone through this process and really understand the biochemistry that is happening with your addictive body response, you will be far better equipped to deal with losing weight than if you try to will yourself into being thin.

A key element in weight loss is the separation of the physical and emotional components of compulsive eating. Compulsive eating, like nicotine use, is a multidimensional process which demands real skill in knowing which factors are motivating you to "use." If you have done the food journal diligently and have gone through each of the food plan steps, you are in a far better place to address your issues around eating. You have learned the power of addiction and have created a whole new way of eating. But if you haven't lost weight, you may be frustrated. Being clear and focused but fat is still no fun. But losing weight will come.

In designing your weight-loss plan, factor in how you will deal with the emotional issues which will come up for you. Geneen Roth does a wonderful job of discussing many of the key emotional issues in her book *When Food Is Love*. Add these principles about feelings to your biochemical skill set and you will be well prepared to start losing weight. I don't agree with her premise that if you allow yourself to eat whatever you crave, you will diffuse the emotional charge in it. My experience, and the experience of all my clients, is that if you continue to eat the foods you crave, you just end up fatter and more miserable. But if you do the emotional work *and* do this food plan, you will improve your chances for long-term success.

In reality, you may have already done much work on the feelings connected to your eating. You may have done thousands of things—diets, seminars, books, groups, therapy, you name it and nothing has held. On the other hand, you may have found that the story outlined in the earlier chapters has given you a new context to understand why it has been impossible to stop your compulsive eating. Most likely, you have already made a significant change in the way you eat. You feel stable, clear and fat. Now you want to feel stable, clear and thin.

Losing weight requires only that you continue the same food plan and move your carbohydrate intake over to the right of the carbohydrate continuum. The further to the right toward green things you go, the more effective your weight-reduction plan will be. This means taking out fruits, juices and brown things for the duration of your weight-loss plan. It does NOT mean taking out carbohydrates and going on a high-protein diet. Most people who are overweight and sugar sensitive have tried the high-protein diet alternatives. They feel wonderful for about three weeks because they have taken all the sugars out and no longer have any beta-endorphin priming. And with less beta-endorphin there will be more beta-endorphin receptor sites. A "little" snack creates a huge response in that upregulated brain and the priming clobbers the diet. Because they are having so little carbohydrate, there will be less tryptophan getting into the brain to make serotonin. Less serotonin also means less impulse control. You are worse off than you were when you started. We all know this pattern. This time, however, you will understand what is happening.

It is essential that you maintain high levels of carbohydrate. But have very, very slow carbohydrates. This means eating lots and lots of vegetables. Counting calories will not work for you. Eating more will. As strange as this seems, eating more vegetables and protein will create an even balance in your brain, reduce the amount of insulin your body releases and facilitate your losing weight. But you have to be particularly rigorous about maintaining every step of the plan.

Let's go through them again:

1. Keep a meticulous journal.
2. Eat three meals a day at regular times and consistent intervals.
3. Maintain your vitamin plan.
4. Eat protein at each meal.
5. Eat only very complex carbohydrates—in this case, green, yellow and red things.
6. Eliminate or drastically reduce all forms of sugars.
7. Create a plan for maintenance.

Use the skills you have developed to design a plan that works for you. Get support. And make sure you eat enough at every meal. Less will not work with this plan. Many people find that having 2 to 3 cups of vegetables and 5 to 6 ounces of protein at each meal works for them. Continue using Mr. Spud at bedtime to maintain the availability of serotonin in your weight-loss process. It may be frustrating that I am not giving you "the diet." You have acquired a great deal of knowledge in the years you did things that did not work or worked for only a short period. By this time I am sure you understand the importance of formulating a plan for yourself. You are the expert. And now, you are the expert with the filter of sugar sensitivity to guide you. Go back to your assessment of your style and re-create a food plan that will create what you want.

Exercise

No book on healing would be complete without a discussion of exercise. Exercise is key to weight loss. The issue is not one of burning more calories but of making your body more sensitive to insulin. You want to move the sugar from your blood into your muscles to be used as fuel. When you are overweight, your body does this less efficiently. Exercise repairs this problem. Exercise also evokes a beta-endorphin response.

Many of my clients have suggested that I include a whole chapter on exercise. But you don't need a whole chapter on exercise. The only thing you need to know is that you have to do it. Exercise is the least complicated part of the equation. *It doesn't work if you don't do it*. And it works if you do. The key is to start. If you are the king or queen of slugs (as I was), the best alternative is to start with 20 minutes a day. Now, for a person who doesn't exercise, the idea of 20 minutes a day may seem overwhelming. But here is a great way to start. In the morning, walk in one direction for 5 minutes, then turn around and walk back. Do the same thing in the evening. You have started with your 20-minutes-a-day plan. If you do this every day for a week, you will find that your body will insist on more. Instead of having to force yourself to exercise, you will find yourself following a body which wants to exercise and is demanding that you keep up. If you continue to be diligent and things do not improve with exercise, then you have more information for your detective story. If you find that you become more and more fatigued rather than energized, check with your doctor about the possibility of having chronic fatigue. This one clue is often a very good pointer to subtle physical illness which will not respond to cranking up the work.

The usual response to exercise is becoming more and more energized and more committed to expanding your program. As your exercise molecules start to sing, you can begin to look at alternatives which suit your lifestyle. You can stroll with your best friend, hike with your children, explore with your dog, Rollerblade, go to the gym, jog along the river, get a personal trainer. If you are overweight,

weight training is an ideal exercise to add to your program. Pumping iron is good for you! It increases your resting metabolic rate and makes your body burn calories faster. Weight training also prevents loss of crucial muscle tissue. Start with the walking and let your body guide you to what you would like to add. But start.

Before long, exercise may become a wonderful part of each day's routine. You will wonder how you ever lived without it. Or you may find that you still don't like it. But do it anyway. Be tender, humorous and simply diligent. In the next chapter you will see why exercise becomes such an awesome part of your recovery.

Chapter 12

Radiant Recovery

Now it is time to start thinking about the long haul. Over time, you may come to feel that this program is too simple. The idea of eating breakfast may seem simplistic and silly. Because there are no sheets and sheets of instructions to be followed, you may presume that this plan isn't really right for you. You may start, do your food journal for a week, get bored with it and decide to go off sugar all at once. A week later you are scarfing up really "healthy" power bars since you know these will give you energy. Of course you feel a whole lot better in the short run. You think you have given up sugar and can lose weight now by eating only two "meals"—a power bar for breakfast, no lunch and then a "healthy" dinner of pasta and salad. Everything seems fine. This plan wasn't for you.

A few months down the road you notice that you are having three double lattes each day, with a bran muffin in the morning, a power bar as a midmorning snack (and later before your workout), pasta salad for lunch and brown rice with vegetables for dinner. You have added two glasses of wine before dinner. Or you may have simply slipped back to having two cups of coffee in the morning on the way to work. Breakfast isn't really that important. And you know that having food will make you fat.

Your energy keeps slipping away, especially in the late afternoon, so you add some more caffeine then to help finish the day. You aren't sleeping too well, but you make no connection to the food you are eating and you assume your fatigue is from job stress. You start getting irritable at work. There's too much to do, not enough time. Your boss is getting on your nerves. You need to stop off for a drink before going home. Weekends bring low-fat, whole grain pancakes instead of the muffin, but much of your days off are spent trying to catch up with your life.

What is wrong with this picture? Your food is low-fat, "healthy." You ask yourself, "Why am I feeling terrible here? Maybe I need to exercise more." You take a "carbohydrate and electrolyte replacement" drink with you to the gym. These drinks are water with sugar and salt. Your energy goes up before the workout, you feel better. Exercise must be the key. But a few weeks later it's not working. What is the matter here? You can hardly get out of bed. You feel as if a truck ran over you.

The answer is simple. Your body is sensitive to sugar. Your blood sugar is spiking up and crashing down all day. You have huge beta-endorphin releases all day (which are causing downregulation and triggering cravings due to priming), and you don't have enough protein to make tryptophan available for conversion into the serotonin you need to do your life. A traditional food plan or "diet" will not provide the answer to your problem.

My solution is simple, but it takes determination to do it. Writing down your food every day requires commitment. You can easily dismiss or forget this step. "I forgot my book," "I went on a trip," "I got busy," "I got bored." Thousands of reasons subvert the process. But your body will remember what it felt like when you ate the way that fits for you. You will now have a molecular memory of what I call radiance. You can always go back to that radiance. The more you can approach this process with humor and appreciation for the long haul, the more you can hang in there with it over time. Most diet plans work for only a short time. The book sits on your shelf, reminding you of yet one more program that sounded good but didn't work for you. This time you are learning skills rather than following sheets of instructions.

Twelve-step programs advise taking life "one day at a time." But when you are in a crisis with your food and you don't feel good, a day is way too long. Take your life *one choice at a time*. Only one choice.

This commitment is all you have to make. Start with breakfast. Make the choice to eat real food for breakfast. Make the choice to have protein. Go back to your food journal. Pay attention to what's happening for you. Find someone to support your process.

Activities to Support Your Radiant Recovery

All through this book you have heard me talk about finding support. I continue to stress this because I know that sugar-sensitive people with their low levels of beta-endorphin have a natural inclination to tough it out. When we are very little, we experience the emotional sense of isolation that comes with low beta-endorphin. So we adapt. We learn to get by on our own. We don't operate from an inherent sense of connectedness to others and we don't realize that this pattern has shaped our way of being in the world. It just seems as if we are busy or shy and we simply don't move well in circles of shared experience.

You have already started moving out of this lifelong pattern by making the biochemical changes that come with changing your food. You may find that now you are open to the idea of support but really haven't a clue how to start. Surprisingly, the answer can be very simple.

You can use existing community resources to support your change. You can go to Weight Watchers, Overeaters Anonymous (OA), TOPS (Take Off Pounds Sensibly), commercial diet programs, or the support group at your local hospital or church. If you choose to go to a program that has prepackaged meals for sale, read the labels. You may find the meals are high in sugar and white flour even though the calories are restricted or balanced. Use your skills. You are an expert detective now. Take the skills you have learned from reading this book and use the strengths of the support plan you have chosen. Some of the ideas I have talked about may contradict what you will learn in these groups, but by now you can trust your own discernment process to sort out what will work for you and what won't.

In fact, the groups themselves may not work for you. You may have tried them and found they don't fit your style or that you are ready for a more dynamic and interactive process. You want a radiant recovery support group. This you will have to create. Talk to people at work or in your neighborhood. Share your process, get people to read this book and talk about their experience. Sugar-sensitive people are lurking everywhere. And we all feel the same way. Ask the chocolate-chip-cookie diagnostic question. Find the cookie lovers. Make a time to get together and share your food journals. In my practice I have a number of people who meet once a week, bring their food journals and talk about how they are doing. The group is very informal and useful. Each person learns helpful ideas from the others. They talk about such subjects as breakfast options or good fast-food choices in the neighborhood. They share hot tips and key ideas.

You may find that your family has a mixed response to your doing this food plan. Initially, they may feel skeptical about your doing "one more diet." When you get to the sugar detox, they may feel horrified that you are going to take away their sugars, too. But as you make changes in the way you eat, you will become more settled, relaxed and energetic. Your family will notice this—the death of Dr. Jekyll and Mr. Hyde will not pass them by—and they are going to want to know what is going on here. Share the power shake. Share the alternatives to simple carbohydrates that you have discovered. You may find they get excited and want to do the food plan with you. Do be careful that in their excitement they don't co-opt your food so you are left without the supplies you need for your own plan.

Or they may decide that they do not want to have anything to do with this plan. They may be incredibly resistant or totally uninterested in anything that has to do with eating more regularly and giving up sugar. They may even actively subvert your commitment to the plan. Your husband may ask, "Aren't you done with that experiment yet?" as he orders a bottle of your favorite wine or takes a big forkful of a dessert that you would kill for. Your kids may come rushing home with a "Mom, look what I brought you!" And they hand you the cookies they know you shouldn't eat, then take them back and eat them in front of you. Remember sugar sensitivity is inherited. Your children may be cookie lovers, too. A close friend who is still very attached to chocolate or French bread may tell you of the dangers of a "high-protein diet." Telling him or her that this food plan is not a high-protein diet will have no impact because the issue isn't really about protein at all. The issue is about resistance to your change. If you change, they may have to. And people in resistance are not ready for change. This is why you need support from people who understand your process and program. Talking with other folks who are supportive is absolutely critical to your success.

Safeguarding Your Progress

Remember the symptoms of relapse so you can be alerted to the vulnerability of the state you are in. Watch for:

- irritability
- fatigue
- general edginess
- thinking that goes round and round
- feeling teary
- emotional fragility
- low tolerance for stress
- inability to concentrate
- feelings of inadequacy

These are the warning signs of relapse. Remember that relapse is not when you consciously have three pieces of chocolate cake. It's when you lapse into unconsciousness and have French bread one day, a bagel the next, a glass of wine the next and then three pieces of cake. Relapse isn't a single event. It's the *process* of losing touch with how vulnerable you are to addiction.

Remember that after you go off a drug for a while, your neuroreceptors upregulate to compensate for the change. If you haven't had sugars for a while, your brain has opened up more beta-endorphin receptors in an attempt to capture whatever beta-endorphin they can. This makes you a sitting duck for relapse unless you pay very close attention. If you have some sugar, you are going to feel fabulous because you now have lots and lots of receptor sites. The sugar you eat will prime the beta-endorphin system and you will start to experience huge cravings. This propels you into a full-blown relapse.

Here's what it can look like:

Karen reports that she had a major slip. She ate a huge piece of chocolate cake. Since then she has had a really hard time getting stabilized. She says she feels as if the floodgates opened and all she wants is sweet things and bread. She sincerely believes the chocolate cake did it.

She goes back to her food journal with a marker and begins highlighting the sugars she had in the week prior to the chocolate cake. The sugar had actually started creeping in about ten days earlier. She was under a lot of stress at work. Someone offered her half a bagel midmorning. She ate it and noted feeling much better, really relaxed. The next evening she went out to dinner and was really hungry so she snacked on French bread before the meal came. She had only "one or two" pieces and didn't think about it at all. The next day she was "hungry" midmorning so she decided to get a cinnamon roll with her decaf coffee at 11 A.M.

She didn't notice what was happening. The following day she felt edgy at midmorning. She attributed it to PMS. After work the kids really got on her nerves. Dinner was running late, they were crabby, she was climbing the walls. The kids came in and got cookies and milk for a snack since she had told them dinner would be late. She felt angry at having to fix dinner anyway. They left the cookie bag on the counter.

Karen poured herself a glass of milk saying, "This is better than drinking wine," and then absentmindedly chomped five cookies while she prepared dinner. The next morning she got up with a headache and felt really edgy. The day was one of high stress on the job. She never got a chance to eat lunch. It was a special occasion so her husband picked her up for dinner. They went to a nice restaurant and had a very pleasant meal. Karen felt ravenous so she ate bread to start, then had pasta with fresh tomatoes and basil.

After dinner she ordered a cappuccino and the waiter with the dessert tray walked by. There in front of her sat a piece of dark chocolate cake with raspberry sauce dribbling over the side. Since this was a special occasion she decided that it would be okay to have the cake "just this once." Karen and her husband had a wonderful evening. She skipped breakfast the next day, had pasta salad on the run for lunch, ate cookies after work and by dinnertime was ready to kill. Her appointment with me came the following day. She woke up then and told me about the slip with the cake at the restaurant.

As I led her through the past week Karen began to see that the cake was really not the slip. In fact there really wasn't an event, there was creeping neurotransmitter interest in the euphoric effect of the sugars. Thousands of upregulated beta-endorphin receptors were just singing at the idea of being stimulated. "More, more!" they were shouting.

The trick to feeling your best is to create a highly balanced system. You do not want a seriously upregulated system. You don't want to prime the little suckers unless you know exactly what you are doing. Unconscious flirtation with sugar-induced euphoria will put you into a very vulnerable place. Your biochemistry will lead you to repeat your actions. Stimulating the beta-endorphin will activate priming. You will feel good and want to do it again. The key here is *paying attention*. Read your food journal, use your yellow highlighter. Know what is happening with your food and your life.

Your goal is not to eliminate sugar for the rest of your life. Your goal is to become aware of what, how and when you eat every day. Going off sugar and changing your food habits is not like going off alcohol, drugs or nicotine. You do not have a day when everything shifts and you become totally abstinent.

If you set yourself up to believe that you will be totally abstinent for the rest of your life, you are simply setting yourself up for failure. Doing a food plan doesn't work that way. It is a *process* of becoming more aware, more attentive, more committed as you go. If you have a cinnamon roll, you need to stop and reflect on what is going on. Listen to your body. Listen very closely. Learn to recognize not only behavioral clues but also emotional and even neurological ones.

Over time, you will come to know the difference between the effects of serotonin decline, beta-endorphin priming and a low blood-sugar reaction. Each has distinctly different symptoms and effects in your body. Your job is to become the leader of the pack. Don't let your impulses take over. Choose your response, your way of dealing with what your body is asking for.

For example, if you find yourself feeling impulsive and irritable, flying off the handle, you are experiencing low serotonin. Have turkey for lunch (for the tryptophan, which goes to make serotonin), then a complex-carbohydrate snack like saltines or Triscuits three hours later. Or crank out ole Mr. Spud at bedtime. Be in service to your healing. Choose the most complex carbohydrate you can so you don't trigger a beta-endorphin spike.

If you feel grumpy and start drifting toward sugar things, go for a vigorous walk to raise your beta-endorphin level. If you feel muddy and unfocused (this can be due to either low serotonin or low beta-endorphin), as if you're in a fog, eat some protein *and* get your body moving.

Living this way will give you confidence and awareness. Rather than being the victim of an inherited body chemistry, you will find joy and delight in your sensitive and complex system. Your inquiring brain will find that food becomes fun and a powerful tool for feeling better and better.

Stopping the Journal

There will come a point when you want to stop keeping your food journal. Assess what lies behind this decision. You may be bored with having to do it—or you may not like what you see. You may be frustrated by your inability to maintain your food plan. If this is the case, continue with your journal anyway, even if you aren't happy about the task.

On the other hand, you may feel you have truly mastered a food plan that works for you and feel you have gone beyond the need to do the journal. Don't stop! Keep doing your journal. You do not go beyond being in relationship to your body. You need to keep paying attention to your eating, though. If your food starts getting sloppy, if your energy changes, if you start getting restless, if you slip into la-la land, if you start to double-book your appointments or forget things and become short-tempered, your journal will be there to help you. Your faithful friend will remind you about your special biochemistry. You may find that your food is stable and that other factors in your life are affecting how you feel. The journal will allow you to either pinpoint factors or exclude them. Either way, you remain a step ahead of the game.

Holding It

As we finish up the dialogue we have had through the course of the book, let's review the key points you want to remember:

Continue your food journal. This book is the cornerstone of your recovery. Doing the journal keeps you *in relationship* to your body. It reminds you of the connection between what you eat and how you feel. The journal keeps you honest and rigorous about what you want. It reinforces living consciously. The journal, as you may have guessed by now, is really about far more than your food.

Maintain your blood sugar level. Stay steady and clear. Always have breakfast. Eat three meals a day at regular intervals. Eat from the right side of the continuum. Stay in good company with brown and green things. Choose foods with the lowest impact value—the least sugars and the most fiber.

Enhance your serotonin level. Eat protein at each meal. Make sure that enough tryptophan is swimming around in your blood. Have a complex carbohydrate (without any protein) three hours after your protein meal to boost little tryptophan into your brain. The baked potato as a nightcap is a powerful tool. Don't be tricked into thinking that this is too simple to work. Pay attention to the effects and you will remain a believer.

Enhance your beta-endorphin level. Reduce or eliminate sugars and white things to minimize the beta-endorphin priming that comes with a hit of sugars. Make life changes to enhance behaviors and activities (listed below) that evoke or support the production of your own beta-endorphin in a steady and consistent way.

Remember that your body was designed for the release of beta-endorphin to support "the good life." Let's list the things besides alcohol, drugs and sugars that evoke beta-endorphin:

Meditation	Prayer
Exercise	Good food
Music	Dancing
Orgasm	Being with the people, puppies or
Listening to inspirational talks	kitties that you love
Yoga	

Most of what's listed have been talked about in the scientific literature. There are scientific articles about the beta-endorphin effect of exercise, meditation, music, yoga, prayer, inspirational talks, sex and palatable food. And no, "good food" does not just mean sugar or fat (although you know those evoke beta-endorphin). Good food means food that tastes good. While the beta-endorphin response to these behaviors is documented in scientific journals, I imagine that your own experience can easily confirm their findings. I added dancing and being with puppies and kitties because the response surely feels like beta-endorphin.

It does seem interesting that the things which are associated with being "high on life" are the beta-endorphin things. It may well be that we were given beta-endorphin to push us to do the things associated with wholeness and happiness.

You may wonder if doing these things will boost your beta-endorphin, create downregulation, then leave you stranded if you can't keep it up. I don't think it works that way. Supporting your body's own production of beta-endorphin with activities like meditation, prayer and exercise enhances the production in a slow, steady rate over time. It does not create those dreaded spikes. So the neurotransmitters and the neuroreceptors stay balanced in the perfect way they are designed to. People who achieve an integrated and focused life, a life with balanced and integrated biochemistry, feel good.

You are learning that the beta-endorphin story is bigger than food.

Discerning Food Issues from Life Issues

After you have followed this plan for a while, you will begin to know clearly and efficiently which physical symptoms *are* connected to your food. Certainly not all of them will be. But the joy for you will be to know how to differentiate. If you are feeling out of sorts you will learn to recognize that your feelings come from a withdrawal from the crazy dessert you had yesterday. The disturbing feelings which are simply part of withdrawal will pass and life will return to normal.

As you have longer periods of time in which your food is stable and clean, you'll also be able to distinguish real-life situations you will need to deal with. Your marriage may be falling apart but you never looked at the reality because you were always medicated with sugar or alcohol. Or your life may not be what you want it to be and you never saw it before because of too many hot fudge sundaes. Or your depression may be creeping back. But you will know so much more about the biochemistry of what is happening, and you will be ready with the options for responding to these issues.

Issues like these are life questions we all must face. There are supports and answers. There are people who can share the journey with you. Discovering these questions will enrich your life and deepen who you are.

There's No Such Thing as Perfection

"Progress Not Perfection" is a core Twelve Step slogan and one that is particularly useful for doing food recovery. You cannot ever have a "perfect" journey with food. Life is too complex and textured for perfection. The real "perfection" you will attain is the joy and confidence you will feel about mastering your "crazy" body chemistry. When I talk about radiance, I am talking about a way of being in the world that reflects your core self. Radiance moves you to humor, tenderness, enjoyment and delight. Radiance urges you to meditate, laugh, dance, pray, sing, paint, read, run, seek good food, intimacy and good company, and connect to meaning. As you step into your new way of being in the world, you will no longer settle for relief from pain or problems. You will want more than that.

You will find that all the work you have done with that funny little food journal has prepared you for taking these next steps, for achieving radiance. The art of paying attention, having a plan and doing one step at a time is an invaluable ally for your future. What you have been practicing these past months is about far more than food. This journey is much bigger than just changing what you are eating. As you heal your food, you are healing the deepest part of who you are. Changing your relationship to food means changing your relationship to yourself, to your nourishment and your connection to your birthright. You are a bright, creative, sensitive and awesome person. These are the benefits of sugar sensitivity.

We've talked a lot about the downside of sugar sensitivity, but the other side of sugar sensitivity is a special kind of awareness, intuition and compassion that comes with the very same biochemistry. Lower beta-endorphin means we are less insulated. We do feel pain more intensely, but we also feel joy more deeply. We know in every part of who we are that something creative, awesome and magical is waiting for us. The same molecules that once sang for sugar will now sing for radiance.

As we come into balance, we can shape our own direction rather than being driven by biochemical circumstances. We feel empowered to make changes in our lives and to control what is happening to us. What seemed like a story about food is really a story about possibility. Fear of being a bag lady or a wino on the street has given way to confidence and opportunity. And it all started with eating breakfast.

APPENDIX A

The Scientific Basis for Sugar Sensitivity

Some people inherit a special body chemistry, called sugar sensitivity, which sets them up to develop specific behavioral and psychological traits. Sugar-sensitive people generally have a family history of alcoholism and are very fond of sweet foods and carbohydrates. They are likely to be impulsive in general, may be compulsive about eating or other behaviors, and may be overweight and/or depressed. They may gain weight disproportional to the amount of calories they consume. They feel both physical and emotional pain more deeply. They may have unexplained or disproportionate anger, overreact to stress and fail to get the results they hope for in psychotherapy. Many have experienced childhood trauma or abuse.

Sugar-sensitive people are often called chocoholics or carbohydrate cravers, or are accused of having a sweet tooth. Their larger-than-normal appetite for sweets or starches doesn't seem to be related to physical hunger. The sugar sensitive eat these foods for emotional reasons or simply to feel comforted. Stressful or highly emotional situations make sugar-sensitive people want to eat even more sweets or breads. Such people may also be very fond of alcohol. Women who are sugar sensitive may be particularly at risk for alcoholic drinking after menopause.

Sugar-sensitive people exhibit strikingly different moods ranging from feelings of wild enthusiasm and competence to despondency and overwhelming hopelessness. These moods can be greatly exaggerated in sugar-sensitive women just before menstruation. In fact, sugar-sensitive people are more likely to be women. Men who are overweight, depressed or impulsive, or who have a particular attachment to alcohol, are also likely to be sugar sensitive.

Sugar-sensitive people may have unexplained physical symptoms which do not respond to traditional medical treatment. These symptoms can include fatigue, restlessness, frustration, irritability, loss of concentration, memory problems, sleep disturbances and headaches.

While not yet scientifically demonstrated, it appears that sugar-sensitive people are likely to be highly creative, exceptionally intuitive and keenly aware of interpersonal dynamics. At times, they may have vivid and powerful dreams. They may also possess extraordinary insight and an ability to quickly come to the crux of complex situations. They may be top performers with a high degree of achievement in their professional lives.

The Science

Let's take a look now at the science underneath the formation of this hypothesis. Sugar sensitivity is a term I have coined to describe those persons who appear to have a dysfunction in three separate but connected biological systems which affect emotions and behavior. These dysfunctions include a disturbance in carbohydrate metabolism, lowered serotonin functioning and a lowered beta-endorphin level which results in an exaggerated response to beta-endorphin-producing exogenous substances. The consequences of these separate disturbances are both physiological and psychological.

Although the hypothesis of sugar sensitivity is inferential at this point, it offers an intriguing possibility of a physiological syndrome which may be identified and examined more fully. The scientific literature has clearly established and discussed extensively the existence of the three problems I have linked together into the syndrome of sugar sensitivity—disturbed carbohydrate metabolism, lowered serotonin functioning and lowered beta-endorphin functioning.

Discussion of the responsiveness to dietary interventions aimed at normalizing these disturbances is prevalent in varying degrees. Data on the resolution of carbohydrate malfunction have been developed extensively and are widely known. Discussion on the role of diet in raising serotonin levels was initiated in the research of Fernstrom at the University of Pittsburgh [1] and Wurtman and Wurtman at MIT [2]. Although these data have not been widely replicated, they have been carefully produced and are well considered within nutritional science. This information has been widely promulgated in the public domain through the popular literature referencing food and mood.

The relevant discussion of beta-endorphin functioning has been found within the alcoholism and addiction literature which has looked at the role of beta-endorphin in the reinforcing properties of alcohol and other drugs. Originally designed as an effective control substance in the beta-endorphin research, sucrose has emerged as an intriguing substance which is consumed for many of the properties it shares with alcohol (i.e., the production of beta-endorphin). The role of sugars consumption as a predictor of human alcohol intake was recently presented in the *American Journal of Psychiatry* [3].

Discussions of the role of diet in the treatment of alcoholism have focused primarily on the development of general restorative diets to enhance nutrient intake and balance blood sugar levels by minimizing the intake of refined carbohydrate products [4, 5]. Other data have suggested the value of increasing sugars intake as a way of maintaining sobriety. The concept of modulating diet as a way of controlling the beta-endorphin priming effects of sugars was first presented in 1996 in my own doctoral dissertation [6]. The concepts presented there have not yet been tested extensively nor replicated in other work.

Disturbed carbohydrate functioning

There has been evidence in both animal and human literature of specific disturbances in carbohydrate metabolism. The working thesis suggests that there are distinct categories of animals and people who are sweet (and alcohol) likers and dislikers, and that these likers and dislikers have different physiological responses to the ingestion of sugar and/or alcohol.

There appear to be distinct and genetically replicable traits for sweet and alcohol preference. Different strains of mice have been bred to be highly drawn to alcohol (C57GL6) or to avoid it (DBA). Rats can be bred to show excessive drinking of sweet solutions [7]. The trait of excessive preference for sweet seems to be particularly sex-linked for the female rats. These rats also show an elevated interest in intracranial self-stimulation [7]. Alcohol-preferring mice also prefer sucrose [8]. The preference for sucrose is not dependent upon prior alcohol intake since the sucrose preference emerges with prior alcohol exposure [9].

Alcohol and sugars seem to have a number of different effects on strains of alcohol-preferring or -avoiding animals. These effects include their response to a sucrose load, the production of insulin, the resistance to the insulin produced and the tendency to obesity. Alcohol has different effects on the carbohydrate metabolism of alcohol-preferring and nonpreferring mice [10]. Alcohol-preferring mice who have never had any alcohol have higher levels of blood glucose in response to sucrose loading than animals bred to avoid alcohol [11]. Alcohol-preferring mice are insulin resistant, and in fact maintain higher levels of baseline insulin from ad-lib feeding [11]. Rats gained more weight from eating sucrose than from eating the same number of calories in other foods [12]. Diets high in simple sugars may produce greater appetite and hunger than diets high in complex starch diets [13].

Although many early studies were done with animals, there is increasing evidence that the same characteristics hold true for humans. Alcoholism and preference for alcohol have been shown to be genetically linked [14]. Certain groups are at risk for alcoholism based on their family history [15]. Alcoholics have also been shown to have a strong preference for sweet foods [16]. A high intake of sweets may predict a motivation for drinking alcohol [3].

A 9 to 17 percent subset of the population are believed to be carbohydrate sensitive. These persons have an exaggerated insulin response to a sucrose load [17]. A combined load of glucose and beta-endorphin also provoked an exaggerated insulin response which was two times higher than the effect of beta-endorphin alone [18]. There appear to be distinct categories of sweet likers and dislikers [19]. Liking and disliking sweets generalizes to sugars other than sucrose [20]. Persons who are tasters of the chemical PTC, 6-n-propylthiouracil (PROP) experience the sweet taste of sucrose more intensely than nontasters [19]. Those persons who had an exaggerated taste response to both sucrose and PROP were classified as "super tasters" [19]. Gender and "self-reported sweet tooth" are highly correlated to differences in alliesthesia (enhancement of sweet taste by hunger) [21]. Carbohydrate cravers have a different response to eating carbohydrates than noncravers. Noncravers are more sleepy, more fatigued and less alert after carbohydrate ingestion than cravers are [22].

The physiological links between liking sweets and craving alcohol have not been studied in the carbohydrate literature. These linkages are discussed more extensively in the alcohol literature looking at beta-endorphin action and will be referenced later.

Serotonin Levels Affect Mood and Behavior

The scientific evidence for the impact of serotonin on mood and behavior is well documented. Lowered levels of serotonin are associated with obesity, carbohydrate craving, depression, impulsivity and violence [23–26]. Lowered levels of serotonin are associated with alcoholism [27]. Persons who have experienced Post Traumatic Stress Syndrome (PTSD) show decreased levels of serotonin [28, 29].

Serotonin synthesis is dependent upon the availability of tryptophan in the blood which can be mobilized into the brain by the ingestion of carbohydrates without concurrent ingestion of protein. The responsiveness of serotonin levels to dietary intervention is also well documented. Brain serotonin increases after ingestion of carbohydrates [22, 30]. Brain tryptophan concentrations and serotonin synthesis are responsive to the sequential ingestion of protein and carbohydrates if there is a sufficient interval between eating [30].

Beta-endorphin Levels Affect
Mood and Behavior

Beta-endorphin is crucial to the sugar-sensitive story. Persons from families at risk for alcoholism have an augmented response to beta-endorphin within the reward systems of their brains [31]. Sugar acts like a drug such as morphine or heroin and evokes a beta-endorphin response [32–36]. Blocking the beta-endorphin receptor sites reduces sucrose intake [35]. The response to the use of sugars can be like the response to other opiate drugs. The motivation to get sucrose increases as the concentration of sucrose does [32]. Sugar use may be considered "the mother of all addiction" [37].

Different people will respond to the druglike effects of sugars in different ways. People with lower levels of natural beta-endorphin will have a heightened response to alcohol, which induces a beta-endorphin response. A moderate dose of alcohol creates a significantly higher beta-endorphin response in persons from families at high risk for alcoholism than in persons from families at low risk for alcoholism. This increased beta-endorphin response is true even when the blood alcohol levels are the same [31]. This augmented beta-endorphin response may extend to the consumption of sugars because of their opioid mediated effects [6].

This heightened vulnerability to the effects of alcohol, opiate drugs and sugars may be particularly true for certain groups, including alcoholics and heroin addicts, who are known to have low levels of beta-endorphin [38], and people from families at risk for alcoholism [39]. Women and overweight persons are also particularly vulnerable to opioid-mediated drugs. There are opiate receptors on the pancreas [18] which may be involved in this reaction. Normal-weight women have lower beta-endorphin than men [40] and respond differently to the opioid modulation of sucrose intake [36]. Because they have less beta-endorphin, women feel pain more deeply than men [41]. Women have even lower beta-endorphin before they menstruate [42]. The drop in beta-endorphin is crucial to the signaling to luteinizing hormone for the preparation of menstruation [42]. Food cravings, physical discomfort and anxiety are associated with the significant decline in beta-endorphin which comes as a result of premenstrual hormonal activity [43, 44]. Chocolate craving peaks in the premenstrual period [45].

Both obese men and women have lower levels of beta-endorphin [40], which appears to play a role in the regulation of appetite [46]. There are opiate receptors on the pancreas and obese men have a significantly higher increase in beta-endorphin after glucose ingestion [47]. This may be a function of a heightened opioid response similar to that of alcoholic men. Obese men may respond to sugars more like women than like normal-weight males who have higher natural levels of beta-endorphin, with concomitantly lower densities of beta-endorphin receptors.

All of these groups (alcoholics and heroin addicts, persons from families at risk for alcoholism, women and obese men) may have shared emotional characteristics as a result of their naturally lowered levels of beta-endorphin. They may experience more learned helplessness [48], have higher levels of separation anxiety [34], have higher levels of loneliness [49], experience emotional and physical pain more deeply [34], and be more prone to tears in the face of emotional distress [49]. They may have less self-esteem, affective hardiness and stability [50]. Because of these emotional deficits, they may seek more isolation, which itself then effects a decrease in opioid peptides [51].

When they use drugs, alcohol or sugars, these persons may also achieve a more powerful relief from the negative physical and emotional states than people who have higher levels of beta-endorphin. The lower beta-endorphin levels create different densities of opioid receptors in their brains [52]. The heightened densities are found in the parts of the brain associated with emotions [52]. Consequently, the experience of emotional stress by these groups may well lead to increased use of opioid-mediating substances [53]. In addition, use of moderate amounts of sugars or alcohol may well prime greater use of the relief-producing substances [54]. Use of some sugars by these groups may well lead to compulsive, long-term addiction [6].

A Solution

Sugar sensitivity describes the presence of these three interactive deficits. The distress created by sugar sensitivity warrants an aggressive intervention. Historically, relief has been sought through intervention aimed at a single phase of the disturbance. However, the complexity of the interactions suggests the value of designing an integrated intervention to address all three simultaneously. The dietary principles outlined in this book address all three of these systems—volatile blood sugar reaction, low serotonin and low beta-endorphin with its concomitant heightened reaction.

The dietary plan stabilizes the blood sugar by normalizing food intake and decreasing the use of insulin-producing foods. It increases insulin sensitivity through dietary change and exercise. The increased insulin sensitivity allows for the emergence of a desired weight more appropriate to caloric intake. It also minimizes negative physical symptoms associated with low blood sugar.

The dietary plan enhances serotonin production by increasing the availability of the serotonin precursor tryptophan through the use of sequential, timed consumption of proteins and carbohydrates. The enhanced serotonin levels are associated with a reduction in carbohydrate craving, sugars use, impulsivity, aggression, depression, compulsive behaviors and alcohol use. They are also associated with an increase in concentration, positive affective states, impulse control, restful sleep and creative action.

Finally, the dietary and life plan reduces the impact of the beta-endorphin priming which comes from compulsive use of alcohol and sugars. Lifestyle changes contribute to the normalization of beta-endorphin function, which can increase tolerance for physical and emotional pain and improve the capacity for isolation. Heightened and stabilized beta-endorphin production appears to enhance self-esteem and affective hardiness, weight loss, emotional stability and creative action. It may also affect capacity to achieve and maintain long-term sobriety.

This protocol, while not yet rigorously studied in a controlled way, appears to have consistent and powerful clinical applications. The dietary and life plan is achieved without invasive action and with minimal side effects. Because it is low cost, easy to learn and highly accessible, it may offer a viable alternative to a pervasive and heretofore intractable problem.

1. Fernstrom, J. D., and R. J. Wurtman, Brain serotonin: Increase following ingestion of carbohydrate diet. *Science*, 1971. 174(Dec. 3):1023–25.

2. Wurtman, J. J., and R. J. Wurtman, Fenfluramine and Fluoxetine spare protein consumption while suppressing caloric intake by rats. *Science*, 1977. 194(Dec.): 1178–80.

3. Kampov-Polevoy, A., J. C. Garbutt and D. Janowsky, Evidence of preference for a high-concentration sucrose solution in alcoholic men. *American Journal of Psychiatry*, 1997. 154(2):269–70.

4. Guenther, R., Ph.D., The role of nutritional therapy in alcoholism treatment. *International Journal of Biosocial Research*, 1983. 4(1):5–18.

5. Mathews-Larson, J., and R. A. Parker, Alcoholism treatment with biochemical restoration as a major component. *International Journal of Biosocial Research*, 1987. 9(1):92–106.

6. DesMaisons, K., Biochemical restoration as an intervention for multiple offense drunk driving. 1996, Ph.D. diss. The Union Institute, Cincinnati, OH.

7. Leibach, I., et al., Morphine tolerance in genetically selected rats induced by chronically elevated saccharine intake. *Science*, 1983. 221(Aug. 26):871–73.

8. Bachmanov, A. A., M. G. Tordoff, and G. K. Beauchamp, Ethanol consumption and taste preferences in C57BL/6ByJ and 129/J mice. *Alcoholism: Clinical and Experimental Research*, 1996. 20(2):201–206.

9. Stewart, R. B., et al., Consumption of sweet, salty, sour, and bitter solutions by selectively bred alcohol-preferring and alcohol-nonpreferring lines of rats. *Alcoholism: Clinical and Experimental Research*, 1994. 18(2):375–81.

10. Forsander, O. A., and A. R. Pösö, Is carbohydrate metabolism genetically related to alcohol drinking? *Alcohol and Alcoholism*, 1987. 1:357–59.

11. Goas, J. A., A. S. Lippa, et al., Endocrine factors underlying the ethanol preference of C57BL/6j Mice. In *Federal Proceedings*, 1978. 37:421.

12. Kanarek, R. B., and N. Orthen-Gambill, Differential effects of sucrose, fructose and glucose on carbohydrate-induced obesity in rats. *Journal of Nutrition*, 1982. 112:1546–54.

13. Geiselman, P., and D. Novin, The Role of Carbohydrates in appetite, hunger and obesity. *Appetite: Journal for Intake Research*, 1982. 3:203–23.

14. Cadoret, R. J., M.D., C. A. Cain and W. M. Grove, M.S., Development of alcoholism in adoptees raised apart from alcoholic biologic relatives. *Archives of General Psychiatry*, 1980. 37(May):561–63.

15. Gianoulakis, C., et al., Different pituitary beta-endorphin and adrenal corti-

sol response to ethanol in individuals with high and low risk for future development of alcoholism. *Life Sciences* (England), 1989. 45(12):1097–109.

16. Yung, L., E. Gordis and J. Holt, Dietary choices and likelihood of abstinence among alcoholic patients in an outpatient clinic. *Drug and Alcohol Dependence*, 1983. 12:355–62.

17. Israel, K. D., et al., Serum uric acid, inorganic phosphorus, and glutamic-oxalacetic transaminase and blood pressure in carbohydrate-sensitive adults consuming three different levels of sucrose. *Annals of Nutrition and Metabolism*, 1983. 27: 425–35.

18. Ipp, E., R. Dobbs and R. H. Unger, Morphine and beta-endorphin influence the secretion of the endocrine pancreas. *Nature*, 1978. 276:190–91.

19. Bartoshuk, L. M., Sweetness: History, preference, and genetic variability. *Food Technology*, 1991. November:108–13.

20. Looy, H., S. Callaghan and H. Weingarten, Hedonic response of sucrose likers and dislikers to other gustatory stimuli. *Physiology and Behavior*, 1992. 52(Aug.):219–25.

21. Laeng, B., K. Berridge and C. Butter, Pleasantness of sweet taste during hunger and satiety: Effects of gender and "sweet tooth." *Appetite*, 1993. 21(Dec.): 247–54.

22. Wurtman, J. J., H. R. Lieberman, and B. Chew, Changes in mood after carbohydrate consumption among obese individuals. *American Journal of Clinical Nutrition*, 1986. 44:772–78.

23. Brown, G. L., M.D., CSF serotonin metabolite (5-HIAA) studies in depression, impulsivity, and violence. *Journal of Clinical Psychiatry*, 1990. 51(4 [suppl.]): 31–41.

24. Virkkunen, M., M.D., Brain serotonin, type II alcoholism and impulsive violence. *Journal of the Study of Alcoholism*, 1993. 11(suppl.):163–69.

25. Hrdina, P., et al., Serotonergic markers in platelets of patients with major depression: Upregulation of 5-HT2 receptors. *Journal of Psychiatry and Neuroscience*, 1995. 20(1)(Jan.):11–19.

26. Wurtman, R. J., and J. J. Wurtman, Brain serotonin, carbohydrate-craving, obesity, and depression. *Obesity Research*, 1995. 3 Suppl. 4:477S–80S.

27. Gill, K., et al., A further examination of the effects of sertraline on voluntary ethanol consumption. *Alcohol*, 1988. 5:355–58.

28. Van der Kolk, B. A., et al., Endogenous opioids, stress induced analgesia, and posttraumatic stress disorder. *Psychopharmacology Bulletin*, 1989. 25(3):417–21.

29. Van der Kolk, B. A., The body keeps score: Memory and the evolving psychobiology of posttraumatic stress, 1993. Massachusetts General Hospital.

30. Fernstrom, M. H., and J. D. Fernstrom, Brain tryptophan concentrations and serotonin synthesis remain responsive to food consumption after the ingestion of sequential meals. *American Journal of Clinical Nutrition*, 1995. 61:312–19.

31. Gianoulakis, C., B. Krishnan and J. Thavundayil, Enhanced sensitivity of

pituitary beta-endorphin to ethanol in subjects at high risk of alcoholism. *Archives of General Psychiatry*, 1996. 52(3):250–57.

32. Cleary, J., et al., Naloxone effects on sucrose-motivated behavior. *Psychopharmacology*, 1996. 176:110–14.

33. Czirr, S. A., and L. D. Reid, Demonstrating morphine's potentiating effects on sucrose-intake. *Brain Research Bulletin*, 1986. 17:639–42.

34. Blass, E., E. Fitzgerald and P. Kehoe, Interactions between sucrose, pain and isolation distress. *Pharmacology, Biochemistry & Behavior*, 1986. 26:483–89.

35. Leventhal, L., et al., Selective actions of central mu and kappa opioid antagonists upon sucrose intake in sham-fed rats. *Brain Research*, 1995. 685(July 10):205–10.

36. Moles, A., and S. Cooper, Opioid modulation of sucrose intake in CD-1 mice: Effects of gender and housing conditions. *Physiology and Behavior*, 1995. 58(Oct.):791–96.

37. Cheraskin, E., M.D., D.M.D., and W. M. Ringsdorf Jr., M.S., D.M.D., A biochemical denominator in the primary prevention of alcoholism. *Journal of Orthomolecular Psychiatry*, 1980. 9(3):158–63.

38. Genazzani, A. R., et al., Central deficiency of β-endorphin in alcohol addicts. *Journal of Clinical Endocrinology and Metabolism*, 1982. 55(3):583–86.

39. Gianoulakis, C., and J.-P. de Waele, Genetics of alcoholism: Role of the endogenous opioid system. *Metabolic Brain Disease*, 1994. 9(2).

40. Ritter, M., et al., Beta-endorphin plasma levels and their dependence on gender during an enteral glucose load in lean subjects as well as in obese patients before and after weight gain. *International Journal of Obesity*, 1991. 15(June):421–27.

41. Gearl, R., et al., Kappa-opioids produce significantly greater analgesia in women than men. Division of Rheumatology, UCSF, 1996.

42. Quigley, M. E., and S. S. C. Yen, The role of endogenous opiates on LH secretion during the menstrual cycle. *Journal of Clinical Endocrinology and Metabolism*, 1980. 51(1):179–81.

43. Bowen, D. J., and N. E. Grunberg, Variations in food preference and consumption across the menstrual cycle. *Physiology and Behavior*, 1990. 47:287–91.

44. Giannini, A., et al., Symptoms of premenstrual syndrome as a beta-endorphin: Two subtypes. *Program Neuropsychopharmacol Biol Psychiatry*, 1994. 18(2): 321–27.

45. Rozin, P., E. Levine and C. Stoess, Chocolate craving and liking. *Appetite*, 1991. 17(3):199–212.

46. Morley, J. E., M.B., B.Ch., and A. S. Levine, Ph.D., The role of the endogenous opiates as regulators of appetite. *American Journal of Clinical Nutrition*, 1982. 35:757–61.

47. Brunani, A., et al., Influence of insulin on beta-endorphin plasma levels in obese and normal weight of subjects. *International Journal of Obesity and Related Metabolic Disorders*, 1996. 20(8):710–14.

48. Besson, A., et al., Effects of morphine, Naloxone and their interaction in the learned-helplessness paradigm in rats. *Psychopharmacology* (Berlin), 1996. 123(1): 71–78.

49. Panksepp, J., R. Meeker and N. J. Bean, The neurochemical control of crying. *Pharmacology, Biochemistry & Behavior*, 1979. 12:437–43.

50. Zorrilla, E. P., R. J. DeRubeis, and E. Redei, High self-esteem, hardiness and affective stability are associated with higher basal pituitary-adrenal hormone levels. *Psychoneuroendocrinology*, 1995. 20(6):591–601.

51. Shoemaker, W., and P. Kehoe, Effect of isolation conditions on brain regional enkephalin and beta-endorphin levels and vocalizations in 10-day-old rat pups. *Behavioral Neuroscience* (U.S.), 1995. 109(1)(Feb.):117–22.

52. de Waele, J. P., K. Kiianmaa and C. Gianoulakis, Distribution of the mu and delta opioid binding sites in the brain of the alcohol-preferring AA and alcohol-avoiding ANA lines of rats. *Journal of Pharmacology and Experimental Therapeutics*, 1995. 275(1):518–27.

53. Van Ree, J., Endorphins and experimental addiction. *Alcohol*, 1996. 13(1): 25–30.

54. Volpicelli, J. R., M.D., Ph.D., et al., Naltrexone in the treatment of alcohol dependence. *Archives of General Psychiatry*, 1992. 49:876–80.

Detoxification from Alcohol

B e tender with yourself as you look at your relationship to alcohol. If you have a problem with alcohol, you probably have had all sorts of people who have been far from tender with you. No doubt you have been criticized, shamed, fought with, talked to, cajoled, bargained with or argued with. In fact, if someone around you criticizes your drinking, it is one of the most reliable indicators that you have a problem with alcohol. People who do not have a problem with alcohol do not evoke pain, frustration or concern about drinking in the people around them.

Take a quiet look at your alcohol use. You don't have to admit you have a problem, you don't have to surrender anything. Your own commitment and experience will guide you in this process. Honesty about your relationship to alcohol is hard because the very nature of the disease of alcoholism is denial. Do this review in the privacy of your own home or office and give yourself absolute discretion over whether you share your findings with anyone at this time. If privacy supports your honesty, embrace it. If sharing serves you better, find a trusted friend to help you ask these questions. The very best alternative is a friend in recovery.

What is very surprising is that people who do not have a problem with drinking don't feel bad about it. They don't feel guilty. We talk a lot about the denial of alcoholism. I believe denial is the response that emerges when people are made to feel defensive about their behaviors. When there is no reason to be defensive, people are remarkably on target about what is going on with them. Take away the shame or the judgment and they can assess their problems pretty clearly.

"Oh, come on," you say. "Everyone does that!" Everyone doesn't do this. People who don't have a problem with alcohol are not inclined to want more when they feel bad. Having a problem with alcohol or alcoholism is defined as "continued use of alcohol despite adverse consequences." When a non–problem drinker has an adverse consequence from drinking, she stops. She will make the connection between feeling bad and alcohol. A problem drinker doesn't see this connection.

Not making the connection is not about being stubborn or stupid or even about willful denial. Not making the connection between drinking and feeling bad is about chemical changes in the brain that alter the parts of the brain that form judgment by making a connection between cause and effect. The parts of the brain that are responsible for saying, "Hey, this made me feel bad. I don't think I want more," don't work properly.

Not making the connection creates a vicious cycle. In the problem drinker's mind, the alcohol actually makes her feel better, so she drinks more. Her opinion is confirmed when the alcohol triggers a beta-endorphin release of euphoric feelings. This reaction is why everyone drinks—the effect is nice. The sugar-sensitive person feels especially good because alcohol causes an even greater beta-endorphin response in her brain. She feels far better than other people do when they drink.

But the next morning she is hung over, a feeling that comes from withdrawal. All the beta-endorphin receptors that were stimulated, or primed, by yesterday's alcohol use are screaming for more. That morning-after feeling of wanting to do *anything* to feel better is so easily taken care of by having a drink. So she does. Relief comes. Blessed, sweet relief. And with her "adverse consequences" switch turned off, the problem drinker's natural response is to feel that having a quick one is a reasonable and logical way to take care of bad feelings. She doesn't know that difficulty with alcohol is creeping up on her.

You may have this same blind spot. How can you know if you have a problem? Let's go back to the questions on page 143. Taken together, these questions form the CAGE, which stands for:

C—CRITICIZED
A—ANNOYED
G—GUILTY
E—EYE-OPENER

Now, let's look at each question individually.

❏ **Have you ever felt you should Cut down on your drinking?** Not a hard one. People usually know the answer to this right away. Yes or no. No cheating or fudging. If cutting down is even a passing thought, answer this one yes.

❏ **Have people ever Annoyed you by criticizing your drinking?** Okay, be honest now. Ever? Think about those times when you held your tongue or wanted to smack someone for making a comment about your drinking. Think of the fights you've had with your spouse about it. Answer honestly.

❏ **Have you ever felt bad or Guilty about your drinking?** This question is pretty straightforward.

❏ **Have you ever had a drink first thing in the morning (an Eye-opener) to steady your nerves or to get rid of a hangover?**

A score of even one is a warning sign about a problem.

Remember the meaning of CAGE. Let yourself think about this for a while. One of two things will happen. You might begin working very hard to say, "Naw, I don't really feel guilty about my drinking." This is an example of denial creeping in and wrapping its deadly little body around your neck. Just pay attention. Consider whether you are getting further away from your relationship to your body and your own inner wisdom.

The other thing that might happen is you may be jostled into realizing that you have a problem with alcohol. If you decide that you would like to stop drinking, there are a number of factors to take into consideration before you do. First, you'll need to estimate how severe a withdrawal you will have based on the frequency and volume of your drinking. You'll need to honestly and accurately figure out how much alcohol you consume in a week. You can do this by recording your alcohol consumption right in your food journal. Do this for a week and then take an honest look at the frequency and amount of your drinking. Calculate the number of drinks you have in a day or a week. A drink is 4 ounces of wine, one beer or 1 ounce of hard liquor. So if you have three 6-ounce glasses of wine (18 ounces), this would be the equivalent of 4.5 drinks.

After you know where you now stand, you can start to plan your detox process. Just as in your detox from sugars, you will want to determine your style for making change. You can either taper down and then stop or you can stop all at once. Most people find it much easier to go for sobriety all at once. You don't have to be making decisions about how much, when, where, with whom all of the time. You can focus on one decision only—the decision not to drink.

It will be important for you to have some sort of support as you make the change. Do not stop drinking without telling anyone what you are doing. Find someone who has been through alcohol detox. Talk to that person. Alcoholics Anonymous (AA) can be a wonderful support because everyone there has been through this process. The only requirement for going to AA is a desire to stop drinking. You don't have to be an alcoholic. You don't have to sign up, you don't have to agree with the program, you don't have to do it any particular way. You don't even have to talk at the meeting. You can sit quietly in the back and slip out quickly anytime you want.

AA can give you a lifeline to others who know about recovery. They can provide you with a road map and concrete suggestions about how to handle what you are feeling. If you go to a meeting and don't like it, don't assume that you won't like a different meeting. Some meetings are boring, some are abusive, and most are profoundly supportive and life-giving.

If you are not comfortable at meetings, find at least one person to support you in your alcohol detox. Do not expect your spouse, partner, daughter or son to be your primary support. They are too closely involved. Find at least one person who has been there. Talk about what you are doing. Tell your story. Get books about recovery. Go to a treatment professional.

If you plan to stop drinking all at once, you must have medical supervision for your detox if any of the following are true for you:

1. If you have a history of blood pressure that is higher than 140/90.
2. If you have drunk more than a six-pack of beer, more than six 4-ounce glasses of wine or more than 8 ounces (half a pint) of liquor daily for over a year.
3. If you have had prior withdrawal symptoms, such as depression or agitation.
4. If you have ever had seizures for any reason, and in particular if you have had alcohol DTs.
5. If you are using any other (either illegal or prescription) drugs in combination with the alcohol. This particularly includes benzodiazepines such as Valium, Librium or Xanax.

Withdrawal from significant or long-standing alcohol use can be a serious process. Keep yourself safe as you make this change. You are taking a very important and brave step. Withdrawal symptoms can include depression, insomnia, sweating, tremulousness, agitation, irritability and brain fog. In fact, go to the sidebar on page 177, which lists the withdrawal symptoms for nicotine. You may experience many of these same things since alcohol and nicotine share some neurochemical pathways. Withdrawal usually starts four to six hours after you usually have your alcohol. If you drink every day at 6 P.M., you will begin to experience discomfort that evening. If you have been a heavy drinker, your doctor may prescribe short-term medication which will minimize the possibility of having seizures during detox.

Making the food changes in preparation for going off alcohol will greatly enhance the likelihood that you can achieve and maintain long-term sobriety. The first week you stop drinking, increase your vitamin and fruit intake. If you feel edgy during the day, have an additional ½ teaspoon of the B-complex liquid. (Don't have it in the evening, though; it will keep you up.) We encourage our clients to have two or three bananas a day for that first week. You can add one to your power shake and then use them as a snack later in the day. Make sure you have a baked potato before you go to bed. It will help your serotonin function and will support the normalization of your sleep patterns.

The clients in my clinic cannot believe what a difference it makes to have done the food plan first. They have fewer withdrawal symptoms, very little craving and feel better than they have in years. This food plan can support the power of your commitment.

Glossary

Abundance model

An approach to healing based on adding rather than taking away. This method helps the individual have a greater sense of possibility, more confidence about options and a sense of hope. The abundance model reinforces the belief that each person knows how to find healing and needs only the appropriate tools to find a healing path.

Addiction

Compulsive use of a substance or behavior characterized by an increasing tolerance for that substance or behavior and the symptoms of physiological withdrawal when the substance or behavior is stopped.

Adrenal fatigue

A progressive physical response by the adrenal glands to long-term stress resulting from difficult situations, the use of alcohol or drugs, or certain dietary patterns, especially the frequent use of sugar. Adrenal fatigue negatively affects the rapidity and effectiveness of the body's normal ability to regulate blood sugar levels and exacerbates addiction.

Antidepressant medications

Psychotherapeutic drugs designed to minimize depression by increasing the availability of serotonin or other neurotransmitters implicated in the physiology of depression.

Beta-endorphin

A brain chemical (specifically, a neurotransmitter) responsible for modulating emotional and physical pain. It contributes to feelings of self-esteem, euphoria and emotional confidence.

"Brown things"

Whole-grain complex carbohydrates retaining high levels of fiber. Includes whole grain breads, whole grain cereals, brown rice, potatoes, lentils, nuts and beans. Go to page 129 for a complete list of brown things.

Carbohydrate continuum

A chart showing the relative complexity of different carbohydrates ranging from simple sugars to wood. See page 118.

Complex carbohydrates

Carbohydrates having more than three simple sugars strung together. Includes starches, brown things and green things.

Covert sugars

Sugars which are hidden in processed foods. Includes high-fructose corn syrup, maltodextrin and raisin paste.

Deprivation model

An approach to healing that requires the individual to give up things. Assumes that the person is unable to make change without rules and restrictions.

Downregulation

A process in the brain by which the number of neuroreceptors for a certain brain chemical decreases to compensate for an increase in the number of neurotransmitters carrying that chemical.

Dr. Jekyll/Mr. Hyde syndrome

The emotional and physical Ping-Pong arising from untreated sugar sensitivity. Feelings and behaviors are erratic and unpredictable, and contribute to greatly decreased effectiveness in dealing with the world.

Endogenous opioids

Neurotransmitters produced within the brain which act as natural painkillers for both physical and emotional pain. Beta-endorphin is a key endogenous opioid.

Food journal

A written log which records the amount and type of food eaten, the date and time, and the physical and emotional feelings of the person keeping the log.

"Green things"

Complex carbohydrates including green, yellow, white, purple and red vegetables. See page 132 for a list of green things.

Hypoglycemia

Low blood sugar resulting from a number of causes, such as not eating regularly or eating foods that are high in sugars. Sugar-sensitive people are more vulnerable to hypoglycemia because they are thought to have an exaggerated insulin response to sweet foods. (See **low blood sugar.**)

Impulse control

The ability to "just say no." The gap between your intention and your action. Mediated by the level of serotonin in your brain. Low serotonin results in low impulse control, and vice versa.

Isolation distress

Emotional pain induced from being separated from a loving and supportive environment. Feelings of isolation distress increase as a person's level of beta-endorphin drops and decrease as beta-endorphin rises.

Low blood sugar

A physical state in which the amount of glucose in the blood drops and creates such symptoms as fatigue, irritability, loss of concentration and emotional vulnerability.

Naltrexone

A drug which blocks the painkilling effect of opioid drugs such as heroin.

Neuroreceptors

Specialized receiving centers on the cell which are coded to accept their matched neurotransmitters and send the appropriate message through the cell.

Neurotransmitters

Brain chemicals responsible for sending specialized messages from one brain cell to another. They include serotonin, beta-endorphin, dopamine and adenosine.

Overt sugars

Sugars that are clearly associated with sweetness, such as table sugar, honey, syrup and the sugars found in ice cream, cookies, cake or soda pop.

PMS

Premenstrual syndrome. A time prior to menstruation in which beta-endorphin levels plummet, cravings for sweets increase, and difficult physical and emotional symptoms are made worse.

Power bar

A nutritional food designed to provide quick energy. Generally billed as low-fat, power bars are often high in multiple sugars.

Priming

The biochemical activation of the beta-endorphin system by one drug, which initiates craving for more of the same or for a drug with a similar effect. For example, eating sugar makes you want more sugar. Eating sugar can also make you want alcohol.

Relapse

A return to compulsive or addictive behavior. See also **slip.**

Reuptake pump

A mechanism that acts like a vacuum cleaner to recycle used neurotransmitters.

Serotonin

A neurotransmitter responsible for mood and impulsive and compulsive behavior.

Simple carbohydrates

Sugars such as the monosaccharides glucose, fructose and galactose, and the disaccharides maltose, sucrose and lactose.

Slip

Short-term flirting with compulsive or addictive behavior. If a slip continues for more than a few days, it progresses into relapse.

Starches

A long chain of hundreds of glucose molecules linked together. Starches are found in grains, beans and vegetables.

Sugar sensitivity

A biochemical condition creating puzzling physical and emotional ups and downs. Sugar sensitivity is characterized by volatile blood sugar responses, a low level of serotonin, a low level of beta-endorphin and a heightened response to the pain-numbing effects of sugars.

Upregulation

A process in the brain by which the number of neuroreceptors for a certain brain chemical increases to compensate for a reduction in the number of neurotransmitters carrying that chemical.

"White things"

Foods made from refined grains and simple starches without fiber. Includes white breads, pasta, white rice and potatoes without the skin. See page 124 for a list of white things.

Withdrawal

A physiological response within the brain when receptor sites have become adapted to a certain level of neurotransmitters and "complain" when that level is reduced. Withdrawal symptoms can include fatigue, irritability, nausea, sleeplessness, headaches, constipation and diarrhea.

Bibliography

Abrahamson, E. M., M.D., and A. W. Pezet, *Body, Mind and Sugar.* New York: Holt, 1951.

Anderson, I. M., et al., Dieting reduces plasma tryptophan and alters brain 5-HT function in women. *Psychological Medicine,* 1990. 20(4): 785–91.

Bachmanov, A A., M. G. Tordoff and G. K. Beauchamp, Ethanol consumption and taste preferences in C57BL/6ByJ and 129/J mice. *Alcoholism: Clinical and Experimental Research,* 1996. 20(2):201–206.

Bagley, R. T., Ph.D., Relationship of diet to physical/emotional complaints and behavioral problems reported by women students. *Journal of Orthomolecular Psychiatry,* 1981. 10(4):284–98.

Barnard, R. J., et al., Effects of a high-fat, sucrose diet on serum insulin and related atherosclerotic risk factors in rats. *Atherosclerosis,* 1993. 100(2):229–36.

Bartoshuk, L. M., Sweetness: History, preference, and genetic variability. *Food Technology,* 1991. November: 108–13.

Bennett, A. E., R. Doll and R. W. Howell, Sugar consumption and cigarette smoking. *The Lancet,* 1970 (May 16):1011–14.

Bertoli, A., et al., Differences in insulin receptors between men and menstruating women and influence of sex hormones on insulin binding during the menstrual cycle. *Journal of Clinical Endocrinology,* 1980. 50:246–50.

Besson, A., et al., Effects of morphine, Naloxone and their interaction in the learned-helplessness paradigm in rats. *Psychopharmacology* (Berlin), 1996. 123(1):71–78.

Blass, E. M., E. Fitzgerald and P. Kehoe, Interactions between sucrose, pain and isolation distress. *Pharmacology, Biochemistry & Behavior*, 1986. 26:483–89.

Blass, E. M., and A. Shah, Pain-reducing properties of sucrose in human newborns. *Chemical Senses*, 1995. 20(1):29–35.

Blass, E. M., and D. J. Shide, Opioid mediation of odor preferences induced by sugar and fat in 6-day-old rats. *Physiology and Behavior*, 1991. 50:961–66.

Bolton, S., Ph.D., G. Null, M.S., and A. H. Pressman, M.S., Caffeine: Its effects, uses and abuses. *Journal of Applied Nutrition*, 1981. 33(1):35–53.

Bowen, D. J., and N. E. Grunberg, Variations in food preference and consumption across the menstrual cycle. *Physiology and Behavior*, 1990. 47:287–91.

Boyd, J. J., et al., Effect of a high-fat-sucrose diet on in vivo insulin receptor kinase activation. *American Journal of Physiology*, 1990. 2(9):E111–16.

Brook, M., Ph.D., and J. J. Grimshaw, B.Sc., F.I.S., Vitamin C concentration of plasma and leukocytes as related to smoking habit, age, and sex of humans. *American Journal of Clinical Nutrition*, 1968. 21(11):1254–58.

Brown, G. L., M.D., CSF serotonin metabolite (5-HIAA) studies in depression, impulsivity, and violence. *Journal of Clinical Psychiatry*, 1990. 51(4 [suppl.]):31–41.

Brown, R., *An Introduction to Neuroendocrinology*. Cambridge, England: Cambridge University Press, 1994.

Brunani, A., et al., Influence of insulin on beta-endorphin plasma levels in obese and normal weight of subjects. *International Journal of Obesity and Related Metabolic Disorders*, 1996. 20(8):710–714.

Bujatti, M., and P. Riederer, Serotonin, noradrenaline, dopamine metabolites in transcendental meditation-technique. *Journal of Neural Transmission*, 1976. 39:257–67.

Cadoret, R. J., M.D., C. A. Cain and W. M. Grove, M.S., Development of alcoholism in adoptees raised apart from alcoholic biologic relatives. *Archives of General Psychiatry*, 1980. 37(May):561–63.

Cerny, L., and K. Cerny, Can carrots be addictive? An extraordinary form of drug dependence. *British Journal of Addiction*, 1992. 87(8):1195–97.

Cheraskin, E., M.D., D.M.D., and W. M. Ringsdorf Jr., M.S., D.M.D., A biochemical denominator in the primary prevention of alcoholism. *Journal of Orthomolecular Psychiatry*, 1980. 9(3):158–63.

Christie, M. J., and G. B. Chesher, Physical dependence on physiologically released endogenous opiates. *Life Sciences*, 1982. 30(14):1173–77.

Chvapil, M., M.D., Ph.D., D.Sc., Effect of zinc on cells and biomembranes. *Medical Clinics of North America*, 1976. 60(4):799–812.

Cleary, J., et al., Naloxone effects on sucrose-motivated behavior. *Psychopharmacology*, 1996. 176:110–14.

Clementz, G. L., M.D., and J. W. Dailey, Ph.D., Psychotropic effects of caffeine. *Journal of the American Medical Association*, 1984. 37(4):167–72.

Cristea, A., A. Restian and G. Vaduva, Endogenous opioid abstinence syndrome. *Romanian Journal of Physiology*, 1993. 30(3–4):241–247.

Cronin, A., et al., Opioid inhibition of rapid eye movement sleep by a specific mu receptor agonist. *British Journal of Anaesthesia*, 1995. 74(2): 188–92.

Czirr, S. A., and L. D. Reid, Demonstrating morphine's potentiating effects on sucrose-intake. *Brain Research Bulletin*, 1986. 17: 639–42.

Dalvit-McPhillips, S. P., The effect of the human menstrual cycle on nutrient intake. *Physiology and Behavior*, 1983. 31:209–12.

de Waele, J. P., K. Kiianmaa and C. Gianoulakis, Distribution of the mu and delta opioid binding sites in the brain of the alcohol-preferring AA and alcohol-avoiding ANA lines of rats. *Journal of Pharmacology and Experimental Therapeutics*, 1995. 275(1): 518–27.

———, D. N. Papachristou and C. Gianoulakis. The alcohol-preferring C57BL/6 mice present an enhanced sensitivity of the hypothalamic beta-endorphin system to ethanol than the alcohol-avoiding DBA/2 mice. *Journal of Pharmacology and Experimental Therapeutics*, 1992. 261(2):788–94.

DesMaisons, K., Biochemical restoration as an intervention for multiple offense drunk driving. 1996, Ph.D. diss., The Union Institute, Cincinnati, OH.

Drewnowski, A., Ph.D., Changes in mood after carbohydrate consumption. *American Journal of Clinical Nutrition*, 1987. 46:703.

Drewnowski, A., and R. C. Greenwood, Cream and sugar: Human preferences for high-fat foods. *Physiology and Behavior*, 1983. 30:629–33.

Drewnowski, A., C. L. Kurth and J. E. Rahaim, Taste preferences in human obesity: Environmental and familial factors. *American Journal of Clinical Nutrition*, 1991. 54(4):635–41.

Drewnowski, A., and C. L. Rock, The influence of genetic taste markers on food acceptance. *American Journal of Clinical Nutrition*, 1995. 62(3):506–11.

Drewnowski, A., et al., Diet quality and dietary diversity in France: Implications for the French paradox. *Journal of the American Dietary Association*, 1996. 96(7):663–69.

Drewnowski, A., et al., Naloxone, an opiate blocker, reduces the consumption of sweet high-fat foods in obese and lean female binge eaters. *American Journal of Clinical Nutrition*, 1995. 61(6):1206–12.

Drewnowski, A., et al., Taste responses and preferences for sweet high-fat foods: Evidence for opioid involvement. *Physiology and Behavior*, 1992. 51(2):371–79.

Dufty, W., *Sugar Blues*. New York: Warner, 1975.

Eades, M., M.D., and M. D. Eades, M.D., *Protein Power*. New York: Bantam, 1996.

Eipper, B. A., and R. E. Mains, The role of ascorbate in the biosynthesis of neuroendocrine peptides. *American Journal of Clinical Nutrition*, 1991. 54:1153S–56S.

Ernster, V. L., Ph.D., et al., Effects of caffeine-free diet on benign breast disease: A randomized trial. *Surgery*, 1982. 91(3):263–67.

Essatara, M. B., et al., The role of the endogenous opiates in zinc deficiency anorexia. *Physiology and Behavior*, 1984. 32:475–78.

Fantino, M., J. Hosotte and M. Apfelbaum, An opioid antagonist, Naltrexone, reduces preference for sucrose in humans. *American Journal of Physiology*, 1986. 251(R):91–96.

Fernstrom, J. D., Ph.D., Acute and chronic effects of protein and carbohydrate ingestion on brain tryptophan levels and serotonin synthesis. *Nutrition Reviews*, 1986. May(suppl.):25–36.

———, Brain serotonin and diet selection. Response to commentaries. *Appetite*, 1987. 8:214–19.

———, Dietary amino acids and brain function. *Journal of the American Dietary Association*, 1994. 94:71–77.

Fernstrom, J. D., and D. V. Faller, Neutral amino acids in the brain: Changes in response to food ingestion. *Journal of Neurochemistry*, 1978. 30:1531–38.

Fernstrom, J. D., F. Larin and R. J. Wurtman, Correlations between brain tryptophan and plasma neutral amino acid levels following food consumption in rats. *Life Sciences*, 1973. 13:517–24.

Fernstrom, J. D., and R. J. Wurtman, Brain serotonin: Increase following ingestion of carbohydrate diet. *Science*, 1971. 174(Dec. 3):1023–25.

———, Brain serotonin content: Physiological regulation by plasma neutral amino acids. *Science*, 1972. 178(Oct. 27):414–16.

Fernstrom, M. H., and J. D. Fernstrom, Brain tryptophan concentrations and serotonin synthesis remain responsive to food consumption after the ingestion of sequential meals. *American Journal of Clinical Nutrition*, 1995. 61:312–19.

———, Large changes in serum free tryptophan levels do not alter brain tryptophan levels: Studies in streptozotocin-diabetic rats. *Life Sciences*, 1993. 52(11):907–16.

———, Protein consumption increases tyrosine concentration and in vivo tyrosine hydroxylation rate in the light-adapted rat retina. *Brain Research*, 1987. 401:392–96.

Forsander, O. A., and A. R. Pösö, Is carbohydrate metabolism genetically related to alcohol drinking? *Alcohol and Alcoholism*, 1987. 1:357–59.

Fredericks, C., Ph.D., *Carlton Fredericks' New Low Blood Sugar and You*. New York: Putnam, 1985.

Free, V., M.A., and P. Sanders, R.N., The use of ascorbic acid and mineral supplements in the detoxification of narcotic addicts. *Journal of Orthomolecular Psychiatry*, 1978. 7(4):264–70.

Froehlich, J. C., et al., Importance of delta opioid receptors in maintaining high alcohol drinking. *Psychopharmacology*, 1991. 103:467–72.

Frye, C. A., and G. L. Demolar, Menstrual cycle and sex differences influence salt preference. *Physiology and Behavior*, 1994. 55(1):193–97.

Gaby, A. R., M.D., and J. V. Wright, M.D., *Nutritional Regulation of Blood Glucose*. 1990, Wright/Gaby Nutrition Institute, Baltimore, MD.

Gearl, R., et al., Kappa-opioids produce significantly greater analgesia in women than men. Division of Rheumatology, UCSF, 1996.

Geiselman, P. J., and D. Novin, The role of carbohydrates in appetite, hunger and obesity. *Appetite: Journal for Intake Research*, 1982. 3:203–23.

Geliebter, A., et al., Effects of strength or aerobic training on body composition, resting metabolic rate, and peak oxygen consumption in obese dieting subjects, 1997. *American Journal of Clinical Nutrition*. 66:557–63.

Genazzani, A. R., et al., Central deficiency of β-endorphin in alcohol addicts. *Journal of Clinical Endocrinology and Metabolism*, 1982. 55(3):583–86.

Gentry, R. T., and V. P. Dole, Why does a sucrose choice reduce the consumption of alcohol in C57BL/6J mice? *Life Sciences*, 1987. 40:2191–94.

George, F. R., and M. C. Ritz, A psychopharmacology of motivation and reward related to substance abuse treatment. *Experimental and Clinical Psychopharmacology*, 1993. 1(1–4):7–26.

Giannini, A., et al., Symptoms of premenstrual syndrome as a beta-endorphin: Two subtypes. *Program Neuropsychopharmacol Biol Psychiatry*, 1994. 18(2):321–27.

Gianoulakis, C., Effect of maternally administered opiates on the development of the beta-endorphin system in the offspring. *NIDA Research Monograph*, 1986. 75:595–98.

Gianoulakis, C., and A. Barcomb, Effect of acute ethanol in vivo and in vitro on the beta-endorphin system in the rat. *Life Sciences* (England), 1987. 40(1):19–28.

Gianoulakis, C., and J.-P. de Waele, Genetics of alcoholism: Role of the endogenous opioid system. *Metabolic Brain Disease*, 1994. 9(2): 105–31.

Gianoulakis, C., B. Krishnan and J. Thavundayil, Enhanced sensitivity of pituitary beta-endorphin to ethanol in subjects at high risk of alcoholism. *Archives of General Psychiatry*, 1996. 52(3): 250–57.

Gianoulakis, C., et al., Different pituitary beta-endorphin and adrenal cortisol response to ethanol in individuals with high and low risk for future development of alcoholism. *Life Sciences* (England), 1989. 45(12):1097–109.

Gianoulakis, C., et al., Endorphins in individuals with high and low risk for the development of alcoholism. In L. D. Reid, ed., *Opioids, Bulimia, and Alcohol Abuse and Alcoholism*. New York: Springer-Verlag, 1990, 229–47.

Gill, K., et al., A further examination of the effects of sertraline on voluntary ethanol consumption. *Alcohol*, 1988. 5:355–58.

Goas, J. A., and A. S. Lippa, et al., Endocrine factors underlying the ethanol preference of C57BL/6j mice. *Federal Proceedings*. 37:421.

Goldman, J. A., et al., Behavioral effects of sucrose on preschool children. *Journal of Abnormal Child Psychology*, 1986. 14(4): 565–77.

Gordis, E., Alcohol and hormones. *Alcohol Alert*, 1994. 26(Oct.).

Gosnell, B. A., and D. D. Krahn, The relationship between saccharin and alcohol intake in rats. *Alcohol*, 1992. 9:203–206.

Grau, J. W., R. L. Hyson and S. F. Maier, Long-term stress-induced analgesia and activation of the opiate system. *Science*, 1981. 213(18):1409–10.

Greden, J., Anxiety or caffeinism: A diagnostic dilemma. *American Journal of Psychiatry*, 1974. 131:10(Oct.):1089–92.

Guenther, R., Ph.D., The role of nutritional therapy in alcoholism treatment. *International Journal of Biosocial Research*, 1983. 4(1):5–18.

Hetherington, M., and J. Macdiarmid, "Chocolate addiction": A preliminary study of its description and its relationship to problem eating. *Appetite*, 1993. 21(Dec.):233–46.

Holt, S., et al., A satiety index of common foods. *European Journal of Clinical Nutrition*, 1995. 49:675–90.

Hrdina, P., et al., Serotonergic markers in platelets of patients with major depression: Upregulation of 5-HT2 receptors. *Journal of Psychiatry Neuroscience*, 1995. 20(1)(Jan.):11–19.

Iny, L. J., et al., The beta-endorphin response to stress during postnatal development in the rat. *Brain Research*, 1987. 428(2): 177–81.

Ipp, E., R. Dobbs and R. H. Unger, Morphine and beta-endorphin influence the secretion of the endocrine pancreas. *Nature*, 1978. 276:190–91.

Israel, K. D., et al., Serum uric acid, inorganic phosphorus, and glutamic-oxalacetic transaminase and blood pressure in carbohydrate-sensitive adults consuming three different levels of sucrose. *Annals of Nutrition and Metabolism*, 1983. 27:425–35.

Jenkins, D. J. A., et al., Slowly digested carbohydrate food improves impaired carbohydrate tolerance in patients with cirrhosis. *Clinical Sciences*, 1984. 66:649–57.

Jias, L. M., and G. Ellison, Chronic nicotine induces a specific appetite for sucrose in rats. *Pharmacology, Biochemistry & Behavior*, 1990. 35(2):489–91.

Kampov-Polevoy, A., J. C. Garbutt and D. Janowsky, Evidence of preference for a high-concentration sucrose solution in alcoholic men. *American Journal of Psychiatry*, 1997. 154(2):269–70.

Kampov-Polevoy, A., et al., Suppression of ethanol intake in alcohol-preferring rats by prior voluntary saccharin consumption. *Pharmacology, Biochemistry & Behavior*, 1994. 52(1):1–6.

Kanarek, R. B., Does sucrose or aspartame cause hyperactivity in children? *Nutrition Reviews*, 1994. 52(5):173–75.

Kanarek, R. B., and N. Orthen-Gambill, Differential effects of sucrose, fructose and glucose on carbohydrate-induced obesity in rats. *Journal of Nutrition*, 1982. 112:1546–54.

Keim, N. L., et al., Effect of exercise and dietary restraint on energy intake of reduced-obese women. *Appetite*, 1996. 26(1).

Kerr, D., et al., Effect of caffeine on the recognition of and responses to hypoglycemia in humans. *Annals of Internal Medicine*, 1993. 119(8):799–804.

Kinsbourne, M., M.D., Sugar and the hyperactive child. *New England Journal of Medicine*, 1994. 330(5):355–56.

Kirkby, R. J., and J. Adams, Exercise dependence: The relationship between two measures. *Perceptual Motor Skills*, 1996. 82(2): 366.

Kuhar, M. J., M. C. Ritz and J. W. Boja, The dopamine hypothesis of the reinforcing properties of cocaine. *Trends in Neurosciences*, 1991. 14(7):299–302.

Kunz, J., Ice cream preference: Gender differences in taste and quality. *Perceptual Motor Skills*, 1993. 77(3 Pt. 2):1097–98.

Kuzmin, A., et al., Enhancement of morphine self-administration in drug naive, inbred strains of mice by acute emotional stress. *Eur Neuropsychopharmacol*, 1996. 6(March):63–68.

Laeng, B., K. Berridge and C. Butter, Pleasantness of sweet taste during hunger and satiety: Effects of gender and "sweet tooth." *Appetite*, 1993. 21(Dec.):247–54.

Leibach, I., et al., Morphine tolerance in genetically selected rats induced by chronically elevated saccharine intake. *Science*, 1983. 221(Aug. 26):871–73.

Leonard, B. E., The comparative pharmacology of new antidepressants. *Journal of Clinical Psychiatry*, 1993. 54(8):3–17.

Leventhal, L., et al., Selective actions of central mu and kappa opioid antagonists upon sucrose intake in sham-fed rats. *Brain Research*, 1995. 685(July 10):205–10.

Lewis, J. W., J. T. Cannon and J. C. Liebeskind, Opioid and nonopioid mechanisms of stress analgesia. *Science*, 1980. 208(May 9): 623–25.

Linnoila, M., M.D., Ph.D., et al., Interactions of serotonin with ethanol: Clinical and animal studies. *Psychopharmacology Bulletin*, 1987. 23(3):452–57.

Looy, H., S. Callaghan and H. Weingarten, Hedonic response of sucrose likers and dislikers to other gustatory stimuli. *Physiology and Behavior*, 1992. 52(Aug.):219–25.

Lowinson, J., P. Ruiz and R. Millman, eds., *Substance Abuse: A Comprehensive Textbook*. 2nd ed. Baltimore: Williams & Wilkins, 1992, 1110.

Macdiarmid, J., and M. Hetherington, Mood modulation by food: An exploration of affect and cravings in "chocolate addicts." *British Journal of Clinical Psychology*, 1995. 34 (Pt. 1)(Feb.):129–38.

Mann, P. E., G. W. Pasternak and R. S. Bridges, Mu 1 opioid receptor involvement in maternal behavior. *Physiology and Behavior*, 1990. 47(1):133–38.

Mathews-Larson, J., and R. A. Parker, Alcoholism treatment with biochemical restoration as a major component. *International Journal of Biosocial Research*, 1987. 9(1):92–106.

Mayfield, D., G. McLeod, and P. Hall. The CAGE questionnaire: validation of a new alcoholism instrument, 1974. *American Journal of Psychiatry*. 31:1121–23.

Mehlman, P. T., Low CSF 5-HIAA concentrations and severe aggression and impaired impulse control in nonhuman primates. *American Journal of Psychiatry*, 1994. 151(10):1485–91.

Melchior, J. C., et al., Palatability of a meal influences release of beta-endorphin, and of potential regulators of food intake in healthy human subjects. *Appetite*, 1994. 22:233–44.

Miller, M., Diet and psychological health. *Alternative Therapies*, 1996. 2(5):40–48.

Moles, A., and S. Cooper, Opioid modulation of sucrose intake in CD-1 mice: Effects of gender and housing conditions. *Physiology and Behavior*, 1995. 58(Oct.):791–96.

Morabia, A., et al., Diet and opiate addiction: A quantitative assessment of the diet of non-institutionalized opiate addicts. *British Journal of Addiction*, 1989. 84:173–80.

Morley, J. E., M.B., B.Ch., and A. S. Levine, Ph.D., The role of the endogenous opiates as regulators of appetite. *American Journal of Clinical Nutrition*, 1982. 35:757–61.

———, Stress-induced eating is mediated through endogenous opiates. *Science*, 1980. 209(12):1259–60.

Moyer, A. E., and J. Rodin, Fructose and behavior: Does fructose influence food intake and macronutrient selection? *American Journal of Clinical Nutrition*, 1993. 58(5):810S–14S.

Muller, B. J., and R. J. Martin, The effect of dietary fat on diet selection may involve central serotonin. *American Journal of Physiology*, 1992. 263(3 Pt. 2):R559–R63.

Naranjo, C. A., M.D., et al., Fluoxetine differentially alters alcohol intake and other consummatory behaviors in problem drinkers. *Clinical Pharmacology and Therapeutics*, 1990. 47(4):490–98.

Niki, E., Action of ascorbic acid as a scavenger of active and stable oxygen radicals. *American Journal of Clinical Nutrition*, 1991. 54:1119S–24S.

O'Malley, S. S., Naltrexone and coping skills therapy for alcohol dependence. *Archives of General Psychiatry*, 1992. 49(Nov.):881–87.

Padh, H., Ph.D., Vitamin C: Newer insights into its biochemical functions. *Nutrition Reviews*, 1991. 49(3):65–70.

Palmer, L. L., Ph.D., Early childhood caffeine and sugar habituation. *Journal of Orthomolecular Psychiatry*, 1977. 6(3):248–50.

Panerai, A. E., et al., Mainly μ-opiate receptors are involved in luteinizing hormone and prolactin secretion. *Endocrinology*, 1985. 117(3):1096–99.

Panksepp, J., Toward a general psychobiological theory of emotions. *The Behavioral and Brain Sciences*, 1982. 5:407–67.

Panksepp, J., R. Meeker and N. J. Bean, The neurochemical control of crying. *Pharmacology, Biochemistry & Behavior*, 1979. 12:437–443.

Pelletier, O., Ph.D., Cigarette smoking and vitamin C. *Nutrition Today*, 1970(Autumn):12–15.

Pennington, J. A., *Food Values of Portions Commonly Used*. Philadelphia: Lippincott, 1994.

Pert, C. B. et al., Neuropeptides and their receptors: A psychosomatic network. *Journal of Immunology*, 1985. 135(2):820s–26s.

Pert C., and H. Dienstfrey, The neuropeptide network. *Annals of the New York Academy of Sciences*, 1988. 521:189–93.

Pierce, E. F., et al., Beta-endorphin response to endurance exercise: Relationship to exercise dependence. *Perceptual Motor Skills*, 1993. 77(3 Pt. 1):767–70.

Pike, R. L., and M. L. Brown, *Nutrition: An Integrated Approach*. New York: Macmillan, 1984.

Pomerleau, C. S., et al., Sweet taste preference in women smokers: Comparison with nonsmokers and effects of menstrual phase and nicotine abstinence. *Pharmacology, Biochemistry & Behavior*, 1991. 40(4):995–99.

Quigley, M. E., and S. S. C. Yen, The role of endogenous opiates on LH secretion during the menstrual cycle. *Journal of Clinical Endocrinology and Metabolism*, 1980. 51(1):179–81.

Rakatansky, H., M.D., Chocolate: Pleasure or Pain? *American Journal of Psychiatry*, 1989. 146(8):1089.

Rappoport, L., et al., Gender and age differences in food cognition. *Appetite*, 1993. 20(1):33–52.

Reid, L. D., and G. A. Hunter, Morphine and Naloxone modulate intake of ethanol. *Alcohol*, 1984. 1(1):33–37.

Reid, L. D., et al., Tests of opioid deficiency hypotheses of alcoholism. *Alcohol*, 1991. 8:247–57.

Ripsin, C. M., et al., Oat products and lipid lowering: A meta-analysis. *Journal of the American Medical Association*, 1992. 267(24):3317–25.

Ritter, M., et al., Beta-endorphin plasma levels and their dependence on gender during an enteral glucose load in lean subjects as well as in obese patients before and after weight gain. *International Journal of Obesity*, 1991. 15(June):421–27.

Rozin, P., E. Levine and C. Stoess, Chocolate craving and liking. *Appetite*, 1991. 17(3):199–212.

Schectman, G., M.D., J. C. Byrd, M.D., and H. W. Gruchow, Ph.D., The influence of smoking on vitamin C status in adults. *American Journal of Public Health*, 1989. 79(2):158–62.

Scheer, J. F., Vitamin C learns some new tricks. *Better Nutrition for Today's Living*, 1992. 54(2):18–21.

Sellers, E. M., M.D., Ph.D., C. A. Naranjo, M.D., and K. Kadlec, B.Sc., Do serotonin uptake inhibitors decrease smoking? Observations in a group of heavy drinkers. *Journal of Clinical Psychopharmacology*, 1987. 7(6):417–20.

Shoemaker, W., and P. Kehoe, Effect of isolation conditions on brain regional enkephalin and beta-endorphin levels and vocalizations in 10-day-old rat pups. *Behavioral Neuroscience* (U.S.), 1995. 109(1) (Feb.):117–22.

Snyder, S., M.D., The opiate receptor and morphine-like peptides in the brain. *American Journal of Psychiatry*, 1978. 135(6):645–52.

Somani, S. M., and P. Gupta, Caffeine: A new look at an age-old drug. *International Journal of Clinical Pharmacology, Therapy and Toxicology*, 1988. 26(11):521–33.

Stewart, R. B., et al., Consumption of sweet, salty, sour, and bitter solutions by selectively bred alcohol-preferring and alcohol-nonpreferring lines of rats. *Alcoholism: Clinical and Experimental Research*, 1994. 18(2):375–81.

Sutherland, G., et al., Naltrexone, smoking behavior and cigarette withdrawal. *Psychopharmacology* (Berlin), 1995. 120(4)(Aug.):418–25.

Terenius, L., Alcohol addiction (alcoholism) and the opioid system. *Alcohol*, 1996. 13(1):31–34.

Tintera, J. W., M.D., Stabilizing homeostasis in the recovered alcoholic through endocrine therapy: Evaluation of the hypoglycemia factor. *Journal of the American Geriatrics Society*, 1966. 14(2):71–94.

Van der Kolk, B. A., The body keeps score: Memory and the evolving psychobiology of post traumatic stress. 1993, Massachusetts General Hospital.

Van der Kolk, B.A., et al., Endogenous opioids, stress induced analgesia, and posttraumatic stress disorder. *Psychopharmacology Bulletin*, 1989. 25(3):417–21.

Vanderschuren, L. J., et al., Mu- and kappa-opioid receptor-mediated opioid effects on social play in juvenile rats. *European Journal of Pharmacology*, 1995. 276(3):257–66.

Van Ree, J., Endorphins and experimental addiction. *Alcohol*, 1996. 13(1):25–30.

Veith, J. L., et al., Plasma beta-endorphin, pain thresholds and anxiety levels across the human menstrual cycle. *Physiology and Behavior*, 1984. 32:31–34.

Virkkunen, M., M.D., Brain serotonin, type II alcoholism and impulsive violence. *Journal of the Study of Alcoholism*, 1993. 11(suppl.):163–69.

———, Reactive hypoglycemic tendency among habitually violent offenders. *Nutrition Reviews*/Supplement, 1986(May):94–103.

————, Serotonin in early onset, male alcoholics with violent behavior. *Annals of Medicine*, 1990. 22:327–31.

Volpicelli, J. R., M.D., Ph.D., et al., Naltrexone in the treatment of alcohol dependence. *Archives of General Psychiatry*, 1992. 49:876–80.

Waterhouse, D., M.P.H., R.D., *Why Women Need Chocolate*. New York: Hyperion, 1995.

Weingarten, H., and D. Elston, Food cravings in a college population. *Appetite*, 1991. 17(Dec.):167–75.

Williams, R. J., Ph.D., Alcoholism as a nutritional problem. *Journal of Clinical Nutrition*, 1952–53:32–36.

Wolraich, M. L., M.D., et al., Effects of diets high in sucrose or aspartame on the behavior and cognitive performance of children. *New England Journal of Medicine*, 1994. 330(5):301–307.

Wurtman, J. J., H. R. Lieberman and B. Chew, Changes in mood after carbohydrate consumption among obese individuals. *American Journal of Clinical Nutrition*, 1986. 44:772–78.

Wurtman, J. J., and R. J. Wurtman, Fenfluramine and fluoxetine spare protein consumption while suppressing caloric intake by rats. *Science*, 1977. 194(Dec.):1178–80.

Wurtman, R. J., Ways that foods can affect the brain. *Nutrition Reviews*, 1986. Supplement(May):2–5.

Wurtman, R. J., and J. J. Wurtman, Brain serotonin, carbohydrate-craving, obesity, and depression. *Obesity Research*, 1995. 3 Suppl. 4:477S–80S.

Yung, L., E. Gordis, and J. Holt, Dietary choices and likelihood of abstinence among alcoholic patients in an outpatient clinic. *Drug and Alcohol Dependence*, 1983. 12:355–62.

Zarrindast, M. R., and D. Farzin, Nicotine attenuates Naloxone-induced jumping behavior in morphine-dependent mice. *European Journal of Pharmacology*, 1996. 298(1):1–6.

Zorrilla, E. P., R. J. DeRubeis and E. Redei, High self-esteem, hardiness and affective stability are associated with higher basal pituitary-adrenal hormone levels. *Psychoneuroendocrinology*, 1995. 20(6):591–601.

Zweben, J. E., Ph.D., Eating disorders and substance abuse. *Journal of Psychoactive Drugs*, 1987. 19(2):181–92.

Resources

Twelve-Step Programs

Most communities have a central office of Alcoholics Anonymous. The staff of this office can guide you to AA meetings or AA members. They can also refer you to other types of meetings more suited to your needs. They will know about:

CA (Cocaine Anonymous)
OA (Overeaters Anonymous)
AlAnon (for families of alcoholics)
DA (Debtors Anonymous)
NA (Narcotics Anonymous)

ACOA (Adult Children of Alcoholics)
CODA (Codependents Anonymous)
SLAA (Sex and Love Addicts Anonymous)

Call local information to get the central office number or call the national office at

212-870-3400

George's Shake

In response to requests from so many of my clients, I have found a company to make a pre-made power shake called George's Shake, which will give you an excellent combination of protein, complex carbohydrates, vitamins and minerals. I will donate my profits from the sale of George's Shake to a nonprofit foundation supporting alcoholism treatment. Call The Vitamin Trader and they can send it directly to your home:

The Vitamin Trader
(800) 344-9310

Newsletter

You can subscribe to the Radiant Recovery Newsletter, *Simple Solutions*, by sending an e-mail to radiantkd@mindspring.com. The newsletter is published monthly and will give you an update on scientific information, helpful hints and resources supportive to your recovery process. There is no charge for the newsletter.

Web Page

Find Radiant Recovery on the Web at www.radiantrecovery.com or e-mail us at admin@radiantrecovery.com. We are delighted to have your feedback and comments. The Web site includes Frequently Asked Questions (FAQs), helpful hints, reviews from people all over the world and a community forum. The Web page also posts our scheduled appearances and lists seminars, talks and other opportunities to meet with us.

Motivational Tools

Tapes

The audio of *Potatoes Not Prozac* is available through the web site at www.radiantrecovery.com or from our office in California. We also have additional tapes to support your process. Topics such as "Getting Started," "The Scientific Evidence" and "Supporting Your Progress" are available on tape.

Support Groups

Support groups are being held in all parts of the country. Check the Web site for locations or call:

Radiant Recovery
1-888-579-3970

Seminars

Seminars are held regularly throughout the country. Seminars are held in many different formats—two hour, all day and weekly. Contact the Web site or the office at 1-888-579-3970 for more information about Seminars.

Books

While I do not necessarily agree with all the recommendations found in these books, I do believe they can provide excellent tools to help you shape your own decision-making process. The more information you have, the more you can discern the path which is right for you.

Abrahamson, E. M., M.D., and A. W. Pezet, *Body, Mind and Sugar*. New York: Holt, 1951.

Beattie, M., *Codependent No More*. Center City, MN: Hazelden, 1992.

Black, C., *It Will Never Happen to Me!* Denver: M.A.C., 1981.

Breggin, P., M.D., *Talking Back to Prozac*. New York: St. Martin's, 1994.

Brown, R., *An Introduction to Neuroendocrinology*. Cambridge, England: Cambridge University Press, 1994.

Cameron, J., *The Artist's Way*. New York: Putnam, 1992.

Carper, J., *Food—Your Miracle Medicine*. New York: HarperCollins, 1993.

Chopra, D., *Perfect Health: The Complete Mind/Body Guide*. New York: Harmony Books, 1991.

Dienstfrey, H., *Where the Mind Meets the Body*. New York: HarperCollins, 1991.

Dufty, W., *Sugar Blues*. New York: Warner, 1975.

Eades, M., M.D., and M. D. Eades, M.D., *Protein Power*. New York: Bantam, 1996.

Ezrin, C., M.D., *The Endocrine Control Diet*. New York: Harper & Row, 1990.

Franklin, J., *Molecules of the Mind*. New York: Dell, 1987.

Fredericks, C., Ph.D., *Carlton Fredericks' New Low Blood Sugar and You*. New York: Putnam, 1985.

Heller, R., M.D., and R. Heller, M.D., *The Carbohydrate Addict's Diet*. New York: Dutton, 1991.

Hoagland, M., and B. Dodson, *The Way Life Works*. New York: Random House, 1995.

Kaiser, J., M.D., *Immune Power*. New York: St. Martin's, 1993.

Ketcham, K., and L. A. Mueller, M.D., *Eating Right to Live Sober: A Comprehensive Guide to Alcoholism and Nutrition*. Seattle: Madrona, 1983.

Kramer, P., M.D., *Listening to Prozac*. New York: Viking, 1993.

Krimmel, E., and P. Krimmel, *The Low Blood Sugar Handbook*. Bryn Mawr, PA: Franklin, 1992.

Lamott, A., *Bird by Bird*. New York: Doubleday, 1994.

Lunden, J., *Healthy Living*. New York: Crown, 1997.

Montignac, M., *Dine Out and Lose Weight*. Los Angeles: Montignac USA, 1991.

Murray, M., and J. Pizzorno, *Encyclopedia of Natural Medicine*. Rocklin, CA: Prima, 1991.

Norden, M. J., M.D., *Beyond Prozac*. New York: Regan Books, 1995.

Northrup, C., *Women's Bodies, Women's Wisdom*. New York: Bantam Doubleday Dell, 1995.

Ornstein, R., Ph.D., and D. Sobel, M.D., *The Healing Brain: Breakthrough Discoveries About How the Brain Keeps Us Healthy*. New York: Simon & Schuster, 1987.

Pert, C., *Molecules of Emotions*. New York: Scribner, 1997.

Pinkola Estés, C., Ph.D., *Women Who Run with the Wolves*. New York: Ballantine, 1995.

Puhn, A., M.S., C.N.S., *The 5-Day Miracle Diet*. New York: Ballantine, 1996.

Robertson, J., *Natural Prozac*. New York: HarperCollins, 1997.

Roth, G., *When Food Is Love*. New York: Dutton, 1989.

Sears, B., Ph.D., *Mastering The Zone*. New York: HarperCollins, 1997.

Slagle, P., M.D., *The Way Up from Down*. New York: St. Martin's, 1987.

Snyder, S., *Drugs and the Brain*, vol. 18. New York: Scientific American Library, 1986, 212.

Somer, E., *Food & Mood*. New York: Holt, 1995.

Waterhouse, D., M.P.H., R.D., *Why Women Need Chocolate*. New York: Hyperion, 1995.

Weber, M., *Naturally Sweet Desserts*. Garden City, NY: Avery, 1990, 238.

Woititz, J., *Adult Children of Alcoholics*. Pompano Beach, FL: Health Communications, 1983.

Wurtman, J., Ph.D., *The Serotonin Solution*. New York: Fawcett Columbine, 1996.

Index

About the Author

Kathleen DesMaisons, Ph.D., a leader in the field of Addictive Nutrition, has been lauded for her identification of the phenomenon of sugar sensitivity as a critical factor in addiction and depression. Dr. DesMaisons is president and CEO of Radiant Recovery, a revolutionary treatment program for alcoholism, drug addiction, depression and self-destructive behaviors such as compulsive overeating and gambling. The program has gained national attention due to its unparalleled success rate and its innovative combination of medical and holistic approaches. Dr. DesMaisons splits her time between the San Francisco Bay Area and Albuquerque, New Mexico.

FOR MORE INFORMATION

My goal is to provide hope and answers for those whose lives have been affected by sugar sensitivity, addiction or compulsive behavior.

If you would like to learn more, please contact us for information regarding seminars, conferences, educational material or consultation.

call toll free: (888) 579-3970
online: www.radiantrecovery.com
E-mail: admin@radiantrecovery.com

Thank you,
Kathleen DesMaisons, Ph.D.